Breastfeeding Best Practices in Higher Education

Michele L. Vancour, PhD, MPH
Michele K. Griswold, MPH, RN, IBCLC

Breastfeeding
Best Practices
in Higher Education

Michele L. Vancour, PhD, MPH,
and Michele K. Griswold, MPH, RN, IBCLC

© Copyright 2015

Hale Publishing, L.P.

1825 E Plano Parkway, Suite 280

Plano, TX   75074

972-578-0400 phone

972-578-0413 fax

800-378-1317 toll-free

www.HalePublishing.com

Library of Congress Control Number: 2014948145

ISBN-13: 978-1-9398474-3-0

Dedication

Michele Vancour:

To my parents, Ron and Joan Vancour, for their unconditional love, unfailing support and sacrifices, which have made so much possible in my life. They helped me realize that dreams do come true.

Michele Griswold:

To my mother, Ginny Kennedy Fortin, for giving me life, showing me how to love and for demonstrating creativity, humor, kindness, tenacity, strength and sacrifice every day of her life. I miss you Mom. To my father, Ron Fortin, for your devotion, care, and support of Mom and the rest of our clan. I love you.

Acknowledgements

Four hungry baby boys gave us our practical introduction, a nurturing foundation, and rewarding breastfeeding lessons. During the early postpartum moments, we realized an intrinsic call to support breastfeeding for all babies. As such, our personal and professional paths led us to explore breastfeeding as a nutritional source, a unique bonding experience for women *and* infants, a natural and sustainable health-enhancing benefit of significant value to women, children and society. We believe that breastfeeding is a woman's gift to herself and to her child. We believe that every mother should have the right to provide milk for her child, and every child should have the right to receive his mother's milk.

It was rewarding to collaborate on *Breastfeeding Best Practices in Higher Education*, and learn about the exceptional practices happening on some university campuses across the country to promote, protect and support breastfeeding.

A huge thank you to Janet Rourke, our editor, Alicia Ingram, and the other amazing talents at Hale Publishing.

We want to thank the chapter authors for telling their stories of lactation support, adhering to timelines, and sharing their trials, tribulations, and successes with us. We are encouraged by the efforts their universities embraced, overcoming diverse obstacles and thriving to provide the best for their breastfeeding students, staff, faculty, and visitors. At the end of the workday, supporting breastfeeding on campus is about supporting families. These authors, often the champions of their own institutions, understand that.

Michele Vancour: I thank the three men in my life — my husband, Pete, and our sons, Nathan and Matthew. They have changed me forever in the best ways imaginable. I thank my parents, who have been my pillars of strength, supporting me throughout the process of writing this book as they have always. I thank my co-workers at Southern Connecticut State University who supported breastfeeding before it was the law. I am grateful to my colleagues and members of the College and University Work-Life-Family Association for sharing their breastfeeding stories. Their journeys and triumphs in providing lactation support on their campuses inspired this book. I also thank the mothers I have met and befriended whose ability to overcome personal and professional challenges to breastfeed their children while working; their perseverance provides validity for workplace lactation support programs. I always will be grateful to my co-editor and friend, Michele Griswold, for believing we could write, edit, and publish this book. She is undoubtedly one of the most brilliant women I know, and a true ambassador for breastfeeding.

Michele Griswold: I thank my husband Matthew. Without him, it would not have been possible to succeed in breastfeeding, either personally or professionally, or anything else for that matter. Thank you to our sons Max and Eli. What does one say about one's children except that I love you both (as big as the sky). I thank my parents and sisters, with love. A heartfelt thanks and shout out to the extraordinary staff (front desk, medical, and nursing) and all of the providers (APRNs and physicians) at Wildwood Pediatrics in Essex, Connecticut. In all my professional years, I have rarely encountered such attention to the provision of skilled, professional, and efficient care, with emphasis on the word "*care*" because they genuinely do. I especially thank Drs. Goff, Burke, Condulis, and DiLorenzo for being pioneers in routine lactation support in the primary care setting over ten years ago. I also thank my mentor and friend and the best nurse ever, Janice Cole RN, IBCLC. I am grateful for the thousands of mothers and children for whom I have had the privilege to provide care. I am certain that I received far more from them than they received from me. I thank my Connecticut Breastfeeding Coalition colleagues, board members, and community partners for their tireless commitment to removing barriers to breastfeeding for Connecticut families. Finally, I thank my mentor, friend, and co-editor, Michele Vancour. Make no mistake, this book was her "baby" and I have felt honored to be given a part. Now, she and I have one more thing that we share.

For additional information and support, please visit our book website: www.academicbreastfeeding.com.

What People Are Saying About This Book

This important volume challenges the notion that higher education is "family friendly" by extending the discussion of breastfeeding away from simple lactation room solutions to a more comprehensive approach of breastfeeding programs. Vancour and Griswold bring together an interdisciplinary group of practitioners and scholars, with over 40 years of experience in higher education, work-life, nursing, and lactation consulting, to provide comprehensive examples of best practice programs and policies with attention to the complexity of breastfeeding programs to include: designing, implementing, funding, and assessing programs. Insights gained from this edited book will be helpful to higher education leaders, human resources professionals, and faculty and staff advocates.

Jaime Lester, Ph.D.
Associate Professor
Higher Education Programs
George Mason University

Michele Vancour and Michele Griswold have assembled a wonderful collection of authors who highlight the outstanding breastfeeding support programs at colleges and universities around the United States. As the book suggests, breastfeeding support programs are an important component of the family-friendly campus and can play a critical role in reducing stress for mothers transitioning back to the workplace. Scholars and practitioners who are interested in implementing similar programs on their campuses will benefit from the wisdom dispensed by these leaders in the field.

Margaret W. Sallee, Ph.D.
Assistant Professor, Higher Education
Department of Educational Leadership and Policy
University at Buffalo

Vancour and Griswold provide a grounding in both public policy and informed practice to assist campus leaders in adhering to excellence in breastfeeding support programs with guidance from leading institutions. Under pressure to comply with the Affordable Care Act, and/or state or local laws that protect a woman's right to express milk, institutions are scrambling to be in compliance.

Moving from mere compliance to fostering win-win scenarios, the editors identify and describe in detail a continuum of best practices in lactation programs for mothers who return to work outside of the home and unto the campus setting.

Jean McLaughlin
Associate Director
American Council on Education (ACE)

Foreword

Thirty-three years ago I faced one of the most difficult challenges of my life—continuing to breastfeed my first baby after returning to work as a university publications director. Although I achieved national awards in the arena of student recruitment campaigns and publications for the university, I failed miserably at what mattered most—meeting my goals for nursing my baby.

As a major department manager with a private office and the ability to set my own schedule, I should have had it easy. It was anything but. The barriers I faced then are unfortunately mirrored today in the experiences of women in nearly every job sector: lack of privacy, unpredictable work schedules, discomfort by co-workers, embarrassment to talk about my needs with my male supervisor, unreliable childcare, and an inefficient milk expression system that made it hard for me to keep up with my baby's needs. A co-worker stepped in to offer her perfect "solution"—free formula from the formula company her husband worked for. He convinced me his product was nearly identical to breastmilk, and I succumbed. As my milk production rapidly waned, I panicked, giving more and more formula until one day I realized that my breastmilk supply had mysteriously disappeared. My goal for a year of breastfeeding would not be met.

While this scenario is all too common among working moms in all industry sectors today, additional challenges complicate breastfeeding for women working in institutions of higher learning. Sprawling campuses, large numbers of staff, fixed class schedules, older buildings with limited space, and varied constituents who need support add layers of complexity. Many women search unsuccessfully for private space to express milk. A time-consuming walk may be necessary to access designated lactation rooms across a large campus. Faculty struggle scheduling milk expression breaks around busy class schedules, and may lack privacy in shared office environments. Women employed in hourly jobs on campus may find it challenging to find privacy or to feel comfortable talking to supervisors about their needs. Students juggle the needs of their nursing baby with class schedules that may not allow for sufficient time to express milk. Visitors to campus may not easily know how to access privacy for milk expression. It is not hard to see why one study found that 80% of nursing women discontinue breastfeeding within their first month back at work following the birth of their baby.[1]

Despite the challenges, the tide in worksite breastfeeding support has made a dramatic shift, and options for support have never been greater. The national Healthy People 2020 goals call

---

[1] Cardenas R & Major, D. (2005). *Journal of Business and Psychology, 20(1):31-51.*

for increasing the number of companies providing lactation support services to breastfeeding employees.[2] In 2011, then U.S. Surgeon General, Dr. Regina Benjamin, launched the historic document, *The Surgeon General's Call to Action to Support Breastfeeding,* calling on communities, employers, and health providers to make breastfeeding easier for new moms. It is hard to put into words the profound pride I felt as I attended the launch and listened to the nation's doctor talk about the importance of employer support for breastfeeding moms, outlining action steps that could make the difference. The nation's *National Prevention Strategy* issued in 2011 also calls for policy changes needed to improve breastfeeding support for employed women.

Both national and state legislation reflect a growing momentum aimed at supporting breastfeeding in the workplace. The Patient Protection and Affordable Care Act, passed in March 2010, amended Section 7 of the Fair Labor Standards Act (FLSA) to require businesses provide nursing women with "reasonable time" and a "private place to express milk that is not a bathroom."[3] The space must be private and free from intrusion from co-workers and the public, and must be provided for up to a year after the baby's birth. Twenty-four U.S. States have passed breastfeeding and employment legislation.[4] Though the provisions of these laws vary widely and not all are as strict as the federal legislation, they nevertheless point to an emerging shift in societal norms for supporting nursing moms in the workplace. Women with children are the fastest growing segment of the workforce today, and they are speaking up in increasing numbers about their needs. As a result, businesses are making changes to adopt policies and practices to standardize lactation support for all employees. In the process, businesses are discovering benefits they may not have anticipated. Supporting nursing women can result in lower absenteeism rates due to improved health by infants,[5] higher retention of their valuable employees,[6] lower health care costs,[7] and improved productivity and morale.[8] Supporting nursing moms at work is, simply, a no brainer. It is a win-win for everyone!

2   U.S. Department of Health and Human Services. Healthy People 2020. (2010). Maternal, infant, and child health objectives. Available online at: www.healthypeople. gov/2020/topicsobjectives2020/objectiveslist.aspx?topicid=26.

3   U.S. Department of Labor, Wage and Hour Division. Break time for nursing mothers. Website: http://www.dol.gov/whd/nursingmothers/

4   National Council of State Legislators. Breastfeeding laws. Website: http://www.ncsl.org/ research/health/breastfeeding-state-laws.aspx

5   Cohen R, Mrtek MB & Mrtek RG. (1995). Comparison of maternal absenteeism and infant illness rates among breastfeeding and formula-feeding women in two corporations. *Amer J of Health Promotion, 10(2):148-153.*

6   Ortiz J, McGilligan K & Kelly P. (2004). Duration of breast milk expression among working mothers enrolled in an employer-sponsored lactation program. *Pediatric Nursing, 30(2):111-119.*

7   Ball T & Wright A. (1999). Healthcare costs of formula-feeding in the first year or life. *Pediatrics, 103(4):871-876.*

8   Galtry J. (1997). Lactation and the labor market: breastfeeding, labor market changes, and public policy in the United States. *Health Care Women Int., 18:467-480.*

HOW to make it work, however, remains a challenge for many. In their 2013 Employee Benefits Survey, the Society for Human Resource Management reported that only 34 percent of companies in the country provide dedicated lactation space, despite federal and state laws, and even fewer (eight percent) provide access to educational resources and support.[9] Employers in all industry sectors, and particularly in non-office settings, report that they need solutions and practical strategies that can work in their unique settings.

Help is now available through resources and initiatives of the U.S. Department of Health and Human Services (HHS). In 2008 I was privileged to develop *The Business Case for Breastfeeding* employment worksite toolkit for the HHS Health Resources and Services Administration's Maternal and Child Health Bureau. This comprehensive initiative provides employers with strategies to implement supportive policies and practices. We conducted interviews with employers across the country in a variety of industries to identify their perspectives and barriers, including lack of space, rigid time schedules, discomfort discussing intimate issues at work, concerns over being fair to all employees, and lack of knowledge about the needs of nursing women. *The Business Case for Breastfeeding* addressed these concerns by providing practical strategies and solutions. The comprehensive turnkey approach targets various levels of business management, including CEOs, human resource managers, wellness coordinators, and supervisors, as well as employees and breastfeeding educators. Thousands of the kits have been distributed to businesses across the country. In addition to the resources, we developed a training curriculum and provided state-based training events in 32 U.S. states. To date, more than 3,000 breastfeeding advocates have been trained to provide technical assistance to businesses. State and local breastfeeding coalitions have worked at grassroots levels to provide help and support for community businesses.

In 2014, the HHS Office on Women's Health built on the amazing success of *The Business Case for Breastfeeding* by launching a national initiative to assist employers of hourly workers and those working in more challenging worksite settings, such as schools, retail stores, restaurants, and manufacturing plants. We began the process by developing partnerships with national business organizations and providing webinars and conference presentations at major business events. Along with Altarum Institute, we worked closely with state breastfeeding coalitions to identify best practices and creative solutions. Our team also traveled to eight states to conduct video interviews with business managers and employees in major industry

---

9   Society for Human Resource Management. 2013 Employee Benefits: Examining employee benefits in a fiscally challenging economy. Alexandria, VA: Society for Human Resource Management.

sectors. Throughout this extensive process, I was truly touched by the resilience of women everywhere who believe passionately in the importance of breastfeeding and persevere through sometimes challenging situations. I was struck by the genuine care and support provided by employers to assure that nursing moms do not have to choose between being a mom and pursuing their careers, and the profound gratitude felt by their employees.

The result of this massive national inquiry was an online searchable resource, *Supporting Nursing Moms at Work: Employer Solutions.* The resource provides hundreds of photos and solutions from 200 businesses representing all industry sectors, along with short videos showcasing personal stories and human-interest perspectives of the value of employee lactation support. The resources, available at www. womenshealth.gov/breastfeeding, include snapshots of numerous colleges and universities with best practices for addressing challenges unique to academia.

National and international organizations are involved in consistent messaging about the need for support. The United States Breastfeeding Committee, which I was privileged to chair from 2012-2013, has included worksite support for breastfeeding women as part of its strategic plan in recent years, and now provides numerous website resources at www.usbreastfeeding.org. Advocacy efforts have been underway for several years to support legislation and policy initiatives that support nursing mothers at work. USBC also provides an online directory of state breastfeeding coalitions, many of whom are trained in *The Business Case for Breastfeeding* and are available to support businesses with implementing lactation support services. During my term as President of the International Lactation Consultant Association in 2010-2012, we were able to launch a Worksite Lactation Support Directory, available at www.ilca.org. This directory lists International Board Certified Lactation Consultants across the world who are trained and skilled in lactation support in the workplace and are available to assist both employers and nursing women returning to work.

A movement has begun!

Academic institutions now have a plethora of solutions to consider for private milk expression spaces, even in the most difficult environments. Designated spaces can be created by converting storage areas and small offices, retrofitting restrooms and shower/locker rooms, and constructing walls in the corner of larger areas. Flexible options when there are fewer numbers of nursing women in a building can include conference rooms, private offices of employees or their managers or co-workers, or erecting screens and partitions to enclose a small area. Childcare centers become a solution for some when nursing women are able to place their infant at the college's child development center. Large campuses may include strategic sites in convenient locations that minimize break time needed to walk to those sites. Campus maps can help employees, faculty, students, and visitors easily identify where private spaces can be found. Campus policies and supervisor training can help assure consistent support for all. Onsite prenatal breastfeeding education and back-to-work classes and consultations with an International Board Certified Lactation Consultant and other community experts help women learn to make it work.

Supporting breastfeeding mothers at work is not hard. It does require creativity to turn spaces into functional lactation rooms, especially in older, established buildings. It requires support at administrative levels and oversight within the wellness, human resources, or other employee benefits divisions. It may require a minimal or a major outlay of funds, depending on renovations that have to be made, but the investment results in a positive return. And it requires partnerships with community resources experienced in worksite lactation support. As more and more institutions make lactation support a priority, more and more options become known.

As the momentum continues to build, the greater question is not just compliance with federal and state laws, but how to achieve a true *culture of support,* particularly within the academic community. How do we move to a society where supporting breastfeeding is simply "what we do," and lactation rooms are as common as water fountains or restrooms in buildings? How do we address disparities and inequities so that all women who are nursing their babies, despite their job settings and roles within the institution, have equal access to support? That's where campus policies come into play, assuring that lactation space is included in new construction, that supervisors are trained and new employees learn about lactation services as part of new staff orientation, that roles and responsibilities of both supervisors and employees are clearly defined, and that access to private space and resources for support is clearly communicated to all constituents.

Academic institutions play a pivotal role in leading the way! As educators of future generations of the work force in all sectors of society, colleges and universities can help normalize what has been a biological norm for women and babies since the beginning of time. Breastfeeding support is not just the law, and it's not just a way to bring about bottom-line benefits. It's the right thing to do.

The time is right! This is an extraordinary time in the history of our country for supporting nursing women at work. National momentum continues to mount, and legislation and policies provide the roadmap. Resources, including this book, help ease the transition to campus-wide support for nursing women, and community partners with expertise in breastfeeding education and support are in place to assist.

Seize the moment! This means going beyond compliance with state and federal laws to creating an environment that values family needs of faculty, staff, and students and normalizes breastfeeding. As one educator put it: "The things that matter most should never be impacted by the things that matter least. Breastfeeding support matters most in the big scheme of things. It's an investment in our staff who are priceless. And we're making a difference."[10]

Cathy Carothers, IBCLC, FILCA
Co-Director, Every Mother, Inc.

---

10 U.S. Department of Health and Human Services, Office on Women's Health. (2014). Supporting nursing mothers at work: employer solutions. Website: www.womenshealth.gov/breastfeeding/at-work

Table of Contents

"Imagine that the world had created a new 'dream product' to feed and immunize everyone born on earth. Imagine also that it was available everywhere, required no storage or delivery, and helped mothers plan their families and reduce the risk of cancer. Then imagine that the world refused to use it."

-Frank A. Oski

Editors' Notes

Michele K. Griswold and Michele L. Vancour

Whether a woman will return to the workplace following the birth of her child is not the question. It is well documented that the majority of women *do* return to work shortly after the birth of their children. In 2008, for example, 56.4% of mothers in the United States participated in the workforce before their children reached one year of age (U.S. Department of Labor, Bureau of Labor Statistics, n.d.). Working mothers face unique parenting challenges associated with separation from their children during work hours. One of these challenges is the continuation of breastfeeding. The separation of mothers and infants in the early postpartum period results in breastfeeding rates that are far below recommended standards for optimal health (Centers for Disease Control and Prevention [CDC], 2013). Subsequently, lower breastfeeding rates in the U.S. population present considerable increased health, economic, environmental, and psychosocial risk, making breastfeeding a favored preventive public health strategy (U.S. Department of Health and Human Services [USDHHS], 2011). Examples of acute and chronic conditions for which breastfeeding provides protection include ear infections, eczema, diarrhea and vomiting, hospitalization for respiratory infections, asthma, type 2 diabetes, sudden infant death syndrome, certain types of cancers, and obesity for children (Ip, Chung, Raman, Trikalinos, & Lau, 2009). For their mothers breastfeeding provides protection from breast and ovarian cancer, and possibly postpartum depression (USDHHS, 2011). Mothers are well aware of the benefits of breastfeeding for themselves and their children across the lifespan and, therefore, the majority of mothers are choosing to breastfeed following the birth of their children. However, the continuation of breastfeeding, should a mother choose to do so, and specifically, the continuation of exclusive breastfeeding remains problematic for the mother who works outside of the home.

Over the past few decades, the historical paradigm of the "stay-at-home" mother has evolved to the point that it is far less common than not. The majority of mothers return to work — 60% of them before their child is six months old (Tuttle & Slavit, 2009). The return to the workplace can be a stressful event. After all, few parents would argue that the birth of a child is, by all accounts, a major life event. In addition to expected stress associated with returning to work, for many mothers choosing to continue breastfeeding, the workplace provides additional stress. Therefore, programs and policies to support families as they transition back to the workplace have focused on areas that tend to ease the adjustment for them, such as providing time and space for mothers to express milk.

These policies and programs benefit families by increasing employee satisfaction (and general life satisfaction by proxy). They benefit employers by decreasing turnover and reducing absenteeism, making family-friendly policies a win-win (Tuttle & Slavit, 2009).

What does it mean to be "family-friendly?" Family-friendly policies are by nature as diverse as families themselves. They are not only relevant to families welcoming a new child, but may also include benefits, such as extended medical leave, for those caring for elder family members. Further, the implementation of family-friendly policies across different employment sectors may be equally diverse, negating a "one-size-fits-all" scenario. However, similarities can be found among like-sectors, and herein lies the benefit of presenting a detailed view of a specific employment sector. In this book we focus on the college and university campus as a unique sector of employment. If you think about it, university campuses are much like small towns or cities. They are their own communities and are largely reflective of the larger community in which they are embedded. To this end, a nice summary of family-friendly policies in the higher education setting appear in a book edited by Lester and Sallee. Published in 2009, *Establishing the Family-Friendly Campus* highlights examples of the implementation of best family-friendly practices among academic institutions in the U.S. This unique volume sparked a shared area of interest by including lactation rooms as a benefit for employed breastfeeding mothers in higher education. In our experience, there appears to be perceived complexity associated with the establishment of breastfeeding-friendly workplace policies in this unique setting. Thus inspired by Lester and Sallee (2009), we chose to expand upon one specific area within the realm of family-friendly policies on college and university campuses in the U.S.—breastfeeding support.

A Policy Matter

Although they may be included among family-friendly practices on campuses, breastfeeding support programs are often discussed in terms of "lactation rooms" and amenities included in those rooms, when, in fact, there are many other factors to consider. Therefore, the editors of this book chose to focus specifically on breastfeeding programs in the higher education setting in order to provide detailed information for those who are considering the implementation of similar programs in this setting. Why breastfeeding? As discussed above, breastfeeding provides substantial benefits to women and children's health and wellbeing, as well as offers significant economic and environmental benefits (Bartick & Reinhold, 2010; Ip et al., 2009; USDHHS, 2011). These benefits will be discussed in greater detail in the following chapter, but the bottom line is: 1.) the majority of mothers initiate breastfeeding; 2.) the majority of these mothers return to the workplace during a time that their healthcare providers recommend breastfeeding for optimal health; and the research is clear that 3.) most mothers discontinue breastfeeding before they intend to (Perrine, Scanlon, Li, Odom, & Grummer-Strawn, 2012). Ultimately, it is also well documented that 4.) the workplace creates a significant barrier to breastfeeding success (USDHHS, 2011). Considering these four factors together provides the rationale for the current trend of lactation programs in the workplace, and the academic sector is no exception. It is critical to note, however, that while supporting breastfeeding employees is indeed a nice item on a family-friendly agenda, another good reason for universities to support breastfeeding is because it is the law.

National public health policy initiatives, such as *Healthy People 2020* (USDHHS, 2010), Section 4207 of the U.S. Patient Protection and Affordable Care Act (ACA) of 2010 (U.S. Department of Labor, Wage and Hour Division, n.d.), *The Business Case for Breastfeeding* (USDHHS, Maternal Child Health Bureau, n.d.; Carothers & Hare, 2010), and *The 2011 Surgeon General's Call to Action to Support Breastfeeding* (USDHHS, 2011) have set objectives for all employers in this area. In addition to federal policies, many state mandates for workplace support of breastfeeding require programming in this area. Additionally, national campaigns, such as "Let's Move," (n.d.) that address childhood obesity, also have contributed to a dialogue regarding breastfeeding in the workplace. Interestingly, while a federal agenda requires employers to support breastfeeding employees, little guidance is offered to help employers to actually implement these programs and policies, raising questions for both employees and employers alike. In other words, employers may know "why" it is necessary to offer programs and policies that support breastfeeding employees, but they may not know "how" to do so in order to be in compliance with the aforementioned mandates.

A Practical Matter

In spite of the paucity of available guidance, in our experience there appears to be a great deal of interest on the part of colleges and universities in learning how to best implement breastfeeding support programs. For example, the College and University Work-Life-Family Association (CUWFA) as recorded in their listserv archives has received repeated inquiries from its members, leading to the creation of a Frequently Asked Question (FAQ) document that is easily accessed on their website. Fortunately for breastfeeding employees, not only are campuses increasingly interested in expanding their services in this important area, they are also eagerly searching for best practices to direct their efforts as they encounter unanticipated challenges in the implementation of their programs. For example, often overlooked among common guidelines is that programs initially planned for employees have the potential to benefit others. On the university campus, an example of an unanticipated challenge may be related to mothers who are students and choose to continue to breastfeed following their return to the campus. Is the student entitled to use "lactation rooms" initially planned for employees? How about visitors to campus?

In this volume we examine the need for workplace support of breastfeeding on the college and university campus, document the best practices in existence across the country, and present demonstrated examples for implementation in the Appendix. Each chapter will focus on a particular campus program or practice supporting lactation and effective components that facilitate planning, designing, implementing, managing, and/or evaluating the initiative. Selected chapters will also address issues around facility usage and planning, budgetary considerations, formation of committees to gain buy-in across campus and facilitate final approvals, and the establishment of quality policies for lactation support. There are undoubtedly many college and universities throughout the United States that are supporting breastfeeding employees on their campuses; therefore, this book doesn't claim to present an all-inclusive list. Rather, it is the editors' intent to present an in-depth picture, as well as highly detailed information regarding the "why" and the "how" a college or university can and should invest resources toward supporting mothers and families in their parenting goals, specifically for infant feeding.

A common theme throughout, leading to the initiation of lactation programs, is compliance with aforementioned laws. In spite of the laws, the reader will notice that many universities regard breastfeeding support to be in line with a system of values that are instilled in their individual missions. To this end, broad and specific barriers to the implementation of programs will be introduced through the experiences of each author. Readers may note that some barriers were shared among several universities and are, therefore, potentially relevant to their own program plans. Examples of shared barriers experienced by many of the universities in this volume and presumably nationwide include funding and space constraints. Therefore, many of the chapters have addressed innovative approaches to solving problems associated with funding and space constraints. The introduction of diverse solutions to common barriers should encourage readers to employ creativity in their own approaches.

Creativity aside, solutions to shared barriers also have some commonalities that emerged serendipitously in the absence of specific guidelines or empiric recommendations. These solutions were "found along the way" and may provide those who are in the early phases of implementation with some anticipatory guidance. One example that was consistently highlighted was the "five-minute walking rule." Several universities that cover a large geographic area stipulate in their policies that rooms for mothers to express milk must be within a five-minute walking distance from their specific place of work or "home base." Needless to say, examples are many and will assist those who are embarking on a plan for this type of program to identify perhaps previously unidentified barriers.

Identification of Best Practices

The following will provide a glimpse of the information that will be found in each chapter. It will be clear to readers that there is a great amount of diversity among programs, both in the genesis of programming and in subsequent implementation. An effort was made by the editors to sample geographically disparate institutions in order to offer readers the opportunity to access information that may be most relevant for their purposes, and perhaps even to provide contact information for further information gathering and potential partnerships.

It will also be clear to readers that innovation and dedication on the part of those leading the efforts, in many cases the chapter authors themselves, was key to the success of lactation support for working mothers in this setting. Finally, it is necessary to add a caveat to the editors' intentions. That is, the best practices identified here cannot possibly be supported empirically, as there is only scant literature pertaining to workplace support for breastfeeding. Similarly, there is even less empirical support for breastfeeding programs in this particular setting. With increased sharing of information, particularly with regard to measures of program outcomes, we are confident that enhanced methods of program evaluation will be forthcoming. The best practices among these programs were identified based on the substantial experience of both editors.

George Washington University (GW), Washington D.C.

Erica Hayton of the George Washington University provides a strong overview of a program that began with an overarching vision. Although some provisions had been in place for breastfeeding employees for some time, the vision for a Breastfeeding Friendly University Project (BFUP) began in 2011 at a breakfast meeting at the home of GW's Provost. The Provost's wife, also an International Board Certified Lactation Consultant (IBCLC), introduced the concept. The result? From a small group of breakfast guests, a committee of more than 100 diverse university-wide partners evolved. Best practices in breastfeeding support at GW are too numerous to list here, but readers will surely be struck by how the overarching vision drove policy creation for this impressive program. One such example was the extension of a typical leave following birth to allow for a longer period of bonding, a critical human-development issue, between mother and infant.

University of Rhode Island (URI), Kingston, RI

Barb Silver, Assistant Research Professor in Psychology at the University of Rhode Island, was instrumental in the establishment of the Work-Life Committee (WLC) at URI in 2003. As a social scientist, Professor Silver and colleagues deliberately constructed the program with a clear philosophical and theoretical foundation. This foundation assumes that supporting breastfeeding on the university campus is not simply a structural response to cultural paradigms, but is essential in order to bring about social changes necessary to meet the demands of the 21st century workforce. That said, there is also attention to structural necessities. As an example, URI's policy requires that new construction on campus must include lactation accommodations. The philosophy of URI's program is clearly woven throughout the pages of this chapter. Best practices in this chapter highlight, among others, the inclusion of breastfeeding support in funding opportunities that aim to advance women in STEM (Science, Technology, Engineering, Math) and in funding to advance early and mid-career scientists.

University of California (UC Davis) Davis, CA

In this chapter Barbara Ashby describes one of the longest-running programs in the country. The UC Davis Breastfeeding Support Program was established in 1995, when few, if any, workplace accommodation laws existed. As pioneers in this area and due to their land-grant heritage, UC Davis's scientific community in human lactation, breastfeeding, and infant nutrition are among the world's most respected and influential researchers in the field. While cutting-edge research disseminates findings that influence infant feeding worldwide, the UC Davis campus Breastfeeding Support Program translates these findings into support for families on campus and within the surrounding community. This chapter describes the Program as a "foundational element" of the University's Vision of Excellence, which is defined in a broad societal context. The Program illustrates, among others, best policy practices that take into account the diversity of families in the support of breastfeeding. As such, benefits are extended to spouses and domestic partners, garnering the support of the Lesbian Gay Bisexual Transgendered Queer (LGBTQ) community and others. Additional innovations consider being "lean, green, and clean" with regard to portable breast pumps and a calculated "five-minute" walking rule.

University of Arizona (UA), Tucson, AZ

Authors of this chapter, Caryn Jung, Janet Sturges, and Darci Thompson provide a detailed overview of UA's Life & Work Connections (LWC) breastfeeding support program. Similar to other chapters, the authors describe the LWC program in the context of the university's mission. In this case, however, the word to describe the broader frame of reference is "lifecourse." This model provides faculty, staff, and students with access to master's level LWC professionals with expertise in early childhood and aging populations, recognizing that life is a continuum and the work environment can and should reflect the needs of individuals across the lifespan. Because of UA's commitment to an integrated and holistic approach to work-life, key partnerships included clinicians at the neighboring medical center. The clinicians give complementary consultations in order to provide faculty, staff, and students with the highest standards of clinical lactation care so that maintaining breastfeeding while on campus is less challenging. Additionally, the lifecourse approach at UA acknowledges that breastfeeding mothers do not stop lactating based on work hours and, therefore, have provided access to lactation rooms 24/7.

Michigan State University (MSU), East Lansing, MI

As described by Lori Strom, MSU served as a "prototype" for nearly 70 other land-grant institutions in the U.S. With a large proportion of women making up their faculty, students, and staff, it stands to reason that MSU began to provide lactation rooms in 1999. Since then the number of lactation rooms in this extensive campus system has grown to nearly 90. This impressive number of rooms can be attributed to a diverse set of interested stakeholders who collaboratively moved the breastfeeding agenda forward by focusing not only on the health benefits of breastfeeding, but also on why these health benefits are beneficial for employers in the form of reduced absenteeism and lower healthcare costs. Consistent with other universities' commitments to research, the breastfeeding support program has provided valuable opportunities for MSU's research science community to formally study the impact that workplace support has on breastfeeding success. This chapter also highlights a technologically savvy approach to lactation room mapping.

Johns Hopkins University (JHU), Baltimore, MD

Last, but not least by far, Michelle Carlstrom, Ian Reynolds, and Meg Stoltzfus highlight breastfeeding support at JHU that was, until 2011, informal and decentralized. The passage of the Affordable Care Act provided an opportunity for JHU to reaffirm and formally augment their commitment to working mothers. In a short time, they have come a long way. In 2011, WorkLife took on the role to coordinate the Breastfeeding Support Program by positioning the Program as an employee benefit within the domain of work and life, and not solely as a room for mothers to express milk. With more than 50,000 employees, JHU integrated the Program into a shared responsibility model that would afford a method of accountability across departments and sectors of the organization. While there is some crossover between universities, such as the "five-minute" rule, JHU has also demonstrated remarkably innovative strategies to meet the needs of such a large employee pool. For example, a vending machine strategically located in JHU's highest volume room provides breastfeeding products and pump accessories, undoubtedly a coup for busy mothers who have perhaps left a critical pump part at home. JHU has also demonstrated a commitment to evaluation strategies that, in turn, provide justification for sustainable program components, such as funding. Tracking the number of visits to the rooms is central to this process. In 2012, JHU documented 18,000 visits to their rooms.

The editors of this book believe that there is perhaps no better example of an issue that is so inherently indicative of the intersection between work and life than breastfeeding. In keeping with this philosophy, breastfeeding provides a solid example of a family-friendly policy that is not only possible to implement, but relatively uncomplicated to implement on college and university campuses. While this book focuses on campuses in the U.S., the information may also have implications for university campuses abroad, given that breastfeeding is a universal health behavior.

Breastfeeding, a preventive health behavior that significantly reduces health risks for an array of acute and chronic diseases for mothers and children, is practiced by a majority of women following birth. This is a health behavior that is also good for the environment in the form of waste reduction from artificial milk storage containers (USDHHS, 2011). If breastfeeding families were able to continue breastfeeding, a marked reduction in healthcare costs would be realized (Bartick & Reinhold, 2010). Mothers are encouraged to breastfeed their children for a minimum of one year by all influential professional health organizations, including the American Academy of Pediatrics (APA; 2012). Unfortunately, an extended duration of breastfeeding is simply not possible for many mothers due to a variety of barriers, most frequently, the workplace setting.

The chapters in this book will help to de-mystify the implementation of breastfeeding policies and programs in the higher education setting. We, the editors of this volume, through our 40 years of combined experience in academia, work-life, nursing, lactation consulting, and coalition leadership, have searched each chapter for best practices. A few of the identified best practices support empirical findings, whereas others are just downright innovative and exhibit a steely resolve on the part of those involved to support mothers and families in their parenting goals. We hope these chapters will assist others in the college and university setting to not only improve their own programs, but to be inspired to create a program where there is none.

Breastfeeding matters to mothers, and mothers make up a large proportion of the country's workforce. Children are our future workforce and our future leaders. Their health is critical and infancy is the period that builds their foundations for life. The editors of this book have had experiences with breastfeeding our own children. We also have experiences implementing breastfeeding policy and practice on the university campus and through state coalition work. The implementation of breastfeeding programs may not be easy, but it is worth the challenges. We hope this book will inspire you to address this critical area of family-friendly policy on your own campuses. We challenge you to "start small," but "think big," as the following programs have done. We encourage you to form partnerships with each other toward solidarity in policies that improve the wellbeing of women in academia and their children, our shared future workforce and leaders.

References

American Academy of Pediatrics. (2012). Breastfeeding and the use of human milk. *Pediatrics, 129*(3), e827-841. doi: 10.1542/peds.2011-3552

Bartick, M., & Reinhold, A. (2010). The burden of suboptimal breastfeeding in the United States: A pediatric cost analysis. *Pediatrics, 125*(5), e1048-1056. doi: 10.1542/peds.2009-1616

Carothers, C., & Hare, I. (2010). The business case for breastfeeding. *Breastfeeding Medicine, 5*(5), 229-231. doi: 10.1089/bfm.2010.0046

Centers for Disease Control and Prevention (CDC). (2013). Progress in increasing breastfeeding and reducing racial/ethnic differences - United States, 2000-2008 births. *MMWR: Morbidity and Mortality Weekly Report, 62*, 77-80.

Ip, S., Chung, M., Raman, G., Trikalinos, T. A., & Lau, J. (2009). A summary of the Agency for Healthcare Research and Quality's evidence report on breastfeeding in developed countries. *Breastfeeding Medicine, 4 Suppl 1*, S17-30. doi: 10.1089/bfm.2009.0050

Lester, J., & Sallee, M. (2009). *Establishing the family-friendly campus*. Sterling, VA: Stylus Publishing.

Let's Move! (n.d.) *White house task force on childhood obesity report to the president.* Retrieved from http://www.letsmove.gov/white-house-task-force-childhood-obesity-report-president

Perrine, C. G., Scanlon, K. S., Li, R., Odom, E., & Grummer-Strawn, L. M. (2012). Baby-friendly hospital practices and meeting exclusive breastfeeding intention. *Pediatrics, 130*(1), 54-60. doi: 10.1542/peds.2011-3633

Tuttle, C. R., & Slavit, W. I. (2009). Establishing the business case for breastfeeding. *Breastfeeding Medicine, 4 Suppl 1,* S59-62. doi: 10.1089/bfm.2009.0031

U.S. Department of Health and Human Services (USDHHS), Health Resources Services Administration (HRSA), Maternal Child Health Bureau (n.d.) *Business case for breastfeeding.* Retrieved from http://mchb.hrsa.gov/pregnancyandbeyond/breastfeeding/

U.S. Department of Health and Human Services (USDHHS). (2011). *The surgeon general's call to action to support breastfeeding.* Washington, DC: U.S. Department of Health and Human Services, Office of the Surgeon General.

U.S. Department of Health and Human Services (USDHHS). (2010). *Healthy people 2020.* Retrieved from http://www.healthypeople.gov/2020/topicsobjectives2020/objectiveslist.aspx?topicId=26

U.S. Department of Labor, Bureau of Labor Statistics. (n.d.). *TED: The editor's desk, Labor force participation of mothers with infants in 2008.* Retrieved from http://www.bls.gov/opub/ted/2009/may/wk4/art04.htm

U.S. Department of Labor, Wage and Hour Division. (n.d.). *Fact sheet #73: Break time for nursing mothers under FLSA.* Retrieved from http://www.dol.gov/whd/regs/compliance/whdfs73.htm

Chapter One
Achieving Breastfeeding Goals for All

Michele K. Griswold and Michele L. Vancour

Breast is Best

Health

Breast is best. Few would argue that a large body of scientific evidence defends the statement that breast is best with regard to the health of women and children. Mothers who breastfeed and infants who are fed their mother's milk reduce their risk for poor health outcomes compared with women who never breastfeed and children who never receive breastmilk. For example, breastfed children have a reduced risk of ear infection, gastroenteritis, severe lower respiratory tract infections, asthma, obesity, diabetes, childhood leukemia, and Sudden Infant Death Syndrome (SIDS). In addition, mothers who breastfeed have reduced risk of type 2 diabetes, as well as breast and ovarian cancers. Early discontinuation (before six months) of breastfeeding or not breastfeeding at all is associated with an increased risk of depression for mothers (Ip, Chung, Raman, Trikalinos, & Lau, 2009). In other words, some breastfeeding is better than none, but for women and children to realize the full potential of breastfeeding, *all* breastfeeding is best for the first six months of a child's life. Because of these significant findings, the American Academy of Pediatrics recommends that infants be fed only their mother's milk (exclusive breastfeeding) for the first six months of life, followed by the addition of complimentary foods and the continuation of breastfeeding for one year and beyond, as mutually desired by mother and infant (AAP, 2012).

Money

Aside from the health-related effects, breastfeeding has substantial economic benefits. One recent study (Bartick & Reinhold, 2010), using similar methodology to an earlier report (Weimer, 2001) estimating a $3.6 billion savings, calculated the direct and indirect costs of ten childhood illnesses, as well as premature deaths that may be avoided, and compared these with 2005 breastfeeding rates and 2007 dollars (an adjustment for inflation). The results were impressive. The authors concluded that if only 90% of families in the U.S. could meet the 2010 objectives of Healthy People 2010 (HP 2010),[11] then $13 billion could be saved annually. Perhaps more compelling, nearly 1,000 deaths may be avoided, most of them children. Maybe 90% seems too high to hope for? The authors also analyzed the cost savings, using the same methodology, if only 80% of families were to meet the national objectives, concluding that $10.5 billion savings could be realized. Either number would be an impressive step in the right direction toward healthcare savings.

Clearly, when cost estimates reach the millions and billions, it can be difficult to make the connection between national healthcare costs and how that may impact an individual family. In light of this, we might also consider the financial impact on families who are either unable to or choose not to breastfeed. Little empiric evidence exists concerning individual costs for formula, however, the *Surgeon General's Call to Action* (SGCTA) (USDHHS, 2011) cites a "$1,200 to $1,500" yearly savings, based on a 1999 report (p. 3). Given the changes in the economy over the past decade or so, it is probably safe to assume that costs are higher than they were in 1999. Also, in the absence of published data, an individual family can likely do a relatively simple calculation for their own budgetary planning purposes. A quick Internet search will provide families with a fair estimate based on the volume or number of ounces their infant consumes per day multiplied by the number of days (six months) and compared with the cost of the selected formula. Needless to say, compared with breastfeeding (which is not necessarily as free as some will claim), formula costs families more.

Environment

What about the cost to the environment? Here again, we have very little published information with which to make environmental impact statements with great confidence. However, as cited by the SGCTA (USDHHS, 2011), "for every one million formula-fed babies, 150 million containers of formula are consumed" (p. 4). This impressive number may or may not accurately reflect the usage of formula containers, but it may offer a start to understanding the practical considerations of formula manufacturing compared with breastfeeding. Aside from the costs associated with formula manufacturing, there are other factors involved by way of fuel in the transportation of formula and subsequent measures of emissions. Also, the marketing of infant formula, discussed in more detail below, may also present another potentially significant impact on the environment in terms of the amount of waste generated. Although there is no research to our knowledge that quantifies the impact that formula has on the environment, it is probably

---

11 The HP 2010 objectives were updated for 2020. HP 2010 only included outcome indicators at six months and 12 months. HP 2020 now includes indicators in exclusivity *and* duration among others.

reasonable to assume that breastfeeding is a "greener" option. A child who is breastfed is the recipient of a clean, sustainable, optimal source of feeding that, aside from a modest increase in caloric intake required by his mother, doesn't generate a lot of trash.

Trends

Breast is best. It would appear that mothers are getting this message based on the trends in breastfeeding data that show a significant increase in the initiation of breastfeeding. That is, the majority of mothers in the U.S. are choosing to breastfeed. Many of them, however, stop before they intended (Perrine, Scanlon, Li, Odom, & Grummer-Strawn, 2012) due largely to societal barriers that will be discussed further below. In short, despite some positive and significant increases in breastfeeding initiation and duration rates across all groups, breastfeeding rates continue to under-achieve national objectives (Table 1.1).

Objectives	% Baseline (2006)	% Target (2020)
Increase the proportion of infants who are breastfed:		
Ever	74	81.9
At six months	43.5	60.6
At one year	22.7	34.1
Increase the proportion of infants who are breastfed exclusively:		
Through three months	33.6	46.2
Through six months	14.1	25.5
Increase the proportion of employers who have worksite lactation support programs	25	38

Table 1.1 Selected Healthy People 2020 Breastfeeding Objectives

U.S. Department of Health and Human Services (USDHHS). (n.d.). *Healthy People 2020. Topics and Objectives, Maternal, Infant and Child Health.* MICH 21-22. Retrieved on January 20, 2014 from http://www.healthypeople.gov/2020/topicsobjectives2020/objectiveslist.aspx?topicID=26

According to the most recent available data on selected racial and ethnic groups, breastfeeding rates in the U.S. are on the rise. The Centers for Disease Control and Prevention (CDC, 2013) report that between the years of 2000 to 2008, the percentage of all infants in the U.S. who were ever breastfed (even once following birth) increased from 70.3% to 74.6%. The percentage of infants who were still breastfeeding at six months increased from 34.5% to 44.4%, and the percentage of infants who were still breastfeeding at 12 months increased from 16% to 23.4%. All data points show remarkable increases within a relatively short period of time. One critical point is that this data is in aggregate form. If we take a closer look at the data, we see very important differences according to race and ethnicity.

For white mothers a significant increase in initiation was reported, from 71.8% to 75.2%. Likewise for those still breastfeeding at six months (38.2% to 46.6%) and at 12 months (17.1% to 24.3%). By way of background, during the past decade or so, even when controlling for factors such as income and education, breastfeeding rates have been persistently lower among black mothers and infants compared with white. It is important to note that although disparities persist, some progress has been made to close the gap among breastfeeding mothers and infants in different groups. For example, from 2000 to 2008, the percentage of black mothers initiating breastfeeding rose from 47.4% to 58.9%. At six months, the percentage of black mothers still breastfeeding increased from 16.9% to 30.1%, and at 12 months from 6.3% to 12.5%. While these data represent significant increases, the prevalence of breastfeeding for black mothers compared with white and Hispanic women warrant attention given the health risks associated with *not* breastfeeding. Finally, significant increases in breastfeeding duration were reported for Hispanic mothers and infants during the same time period. In 2008, the percentage of Hispanic women initiating breastfeeding was 80%, an increase from 77.6% in 2000. For breastfeeding duration Hispanic mothers showed significant increases at six months and at 12 months—34.6% to 45.2% and 18.2% to 26.3%, respectively (CDC, 2013). The methodology involved in data collection and its subsequent limitations is beyond the scope of this chapter and book; however, the data cited here is among the best available to date.

Breast is best. Or is it? Frankly, breastfeeding practices and, moreover, racial and ethnic differences in breastfeeding practices are just downright complex. Nevertheless, the phrase "breast is best" seems to resonate with the majority of mothers. Even though the phrase may resonate, it also presents a very high standard for parents who may find little consolation in knowing they "tried," but were forced to discontinue before they intended due to circumstances beyond their control. In summary, the good news for public health is that mothers seem to agree that breast is best, as most women initiate breastfeeding upon the birth of their infants. The bad news for public health is that changing societal norms to reflect an accepting and accommodating culture is proving to be a difficult task, leaving one to wonder if breast is only best under the best of circumstances. That may be the case.

Making Breastfeeding Work

The obvious question is "why is it so difficult to continue breastfeeding?" The answers are anything but simple. In 2011, the office of the United States Surgeon General released a report entitled *The Surgeon General's Call to Action to Support Breastfeeding* (USDHHS, 2011). The report was the first from the office of the Surgeon General since the landmark release of the *Surgeon General's Workshop on Breastfeeding* in 1984 (Galson, 2009). What made the 2011 report so noteworthy was that it called on everyone in the nation to support breastfeeding mothers within their sector of society, and further, it provided concrete action steps that could be taken to support breastfeeding within each sector. The six sectors of society defined by the report are as follows: Mothers and their Families, Communities, Health Care, Employment, Research and Surveillance, and Public Health Infrastructure (USDHHS, 2011). The report also summarized the salient research on the barriers that prevent mothers from reaching their breastfeeding goals. These are as follows: lack of knowledge, social norms, poor family and societal support, embarrassment, lactation problems, employment and childcare, and barriers related to health services (USDHHS, 2011). Each of these barriers represents multi-faceted, complex systems and, therefore, the interventions suggested by the report target multiple levels of influence concerning the nursing mother. It is important to recognize that neither the boundaries between sectors, nor the boundaries between barriers are clearly delineated, but, rather, are interrelated. However, for the purposes of this chapter, we will focus on the employment sector and the associated barriers that mothers may face when choosing to combine work with breastfeeding.

Employment Barriers

As discussed previously, the majority of mothers return to work (56.4%), and 60% of them return before their child is six months (U.S. Department of Labor, Bureau of Labor Statistics, 2009; Tuttle & Slavit, 2009). The return to the workplace following birth can be a stressful event for parents of infants, and there are many considerations, beginning with infant care. One of the most important considerations for the care of infants is how they will be fed and with good reason. As discussed previously, breastfeeding is consistently favored over artificial feeding due to the myriad of benefits associated with the behavior (Ip et al., 2009; USDHHS, 2011), and most women are choosing to breastfeed (CDC, 2013). What is less clear than the decision to breastfeed or not is how to actually make breastfeeding "work" when returning to work. To that end, there are a number of considerations for parents. For starters, women must consider how to express milk while they are away from their infants in order to continue to produce enough milk. For most, this entails using some type of mechanical breast pump. Another consideration close to the top of the list is how often she will need to express milk during the workday, followed by how much time each "pumping break" will take. Next, is there a place to store her expressed milk? "How much milk will my baby need for each feeding?" "What do I do if my baby won't take a bottle?" From there, a seemingly infinite number of questions may arise, such as, "Is there a private place or space to pump?" and "What do I do if I have to travel?" These types of questions lead to some barriers that may be associated with specific work environments.

For women in positions that afford some flexibility, the aforementioned concerns may not be insurmountable. For example, if a woman has her own private office with a lock on the door, some of the questions can be eliminated. Likewise, if a mother earns a salary, then whether or not she will be paid for break time may not be an issue. However, for many mothers who return to the workplace following birth, these problems do not have simple solutions, leading one to perhaps gain some insight into the disparities associated with the continuation of breastfeeding for say, women in lower income categories (CDC, 2013). To that end, let's consider some of the questions that may be pertinent to women who may be paid by the hour and are not salaried employees. "How can I pay for a breast pump?" and "If I take unpaid breaks to pump, then will my number of hours worked be too low to keep my insurance?" A short case study might be helpful here. Let's use the example of a woman who works in a factory and is paid by quota, or the number of pieces that she assembles. Taking unpaid breaks to pump decreases her productivity on the line and subsequently her weekly paycheck. For parents who are barely making ends meet, having to trade future health benefits for keeping the lights on, not only seems reasonable, it seems like a matter of survival. Readers who are mothers and parents can probably relate to the thought processes that quickly unfold in anticipation of returning to the workplace following maternity leave, and we haven't even begun to address the infant's needs where breastfeeding is concerned.

So what does all this mean for mothers who plan to return to work following the birth of their infants? The SGCTA (USDHHS, 2011) summarizes the large and growing body of research that sheds some light on this question. It will come as no surprise that women who are employed outside of the home generally initiate breastfeeding (start breastfeeding right after birth) at lower rates than mothers who are not employed outside the home. Mothers who do initiate breastfeeding tend to have shorter duration (stop breastfeeding before they intended to or before it is recommended). The factors that appear to increase breastfeeding success include a longer period of leave following birth, flexible working hours, such as part-time options, and breastfeeding support programs in the workplace. These factors will be important to keep in mind when reading the following chapters regarding lactation support in selected universities.

Employment Data

Generally speaking, the employment sector is a barrier to breastfeeding in and of itself based on the fact that mothers and their infants will be separated from one another for long periods of time. In addition, as highlighted above, there are many other barriers that are highly specific to individual employment settings, and they vary widely from one worksite to another. Currently, no randomized controlled trials exist that aim to measure workplace interventions that improve breastfeeding success (Abdulwadud & Snow, 2012), but that doesn't mean we cannot glean some important information from other sources of information.

One widely cited source of information with regard to workplace lactation accommodations comes from an annual survey conducted by the Society Human Resource Management ([SHRM]; 2013). The SHRM is an organization of approximately 260,000 diverse businesses across sectors too many to name. Some examples of the broad categories of membership are Healthcare, Finance and Insurance, Retail and Trade, and Educational Services, which include primary and secondary education, as well as post-secondary institutions. The survey also covers broad categories of benefits, one being "Family Friendly" benefits. The questions regarding lactation support fall under this category. A summary of the survey methodology and salient findings follows.

The 2013 SHRM survey randomly sampled 4,000 Human Resource members through email. Among the 3,600 emails that were delivered, there was a 14% response rate. Results indicated that in 2013, 34% of SHRM members had an on-site lactation or mother's room. What does this tell us? First, this represents an increase from the 2009 survey that reported only 25% of worksites with lactation support. Next, it may also tell us that progress is being made toward meeting the objective of HP 2020 to increase the proportion of employers who have lactation support services (see Table 1.1).

What doesn't it tell us? Simply put, it doesn't tell us (for the purposes of this book) the number, if any, of college and universities that represent the nine percent of respondents from the Educational Services setting. It also doesn't tell us if this is a statistically significant increase. Because of the way the survey question regarding lactation rooms is worded, "a separate room that goes above and beyond the requirements of the ACA" (SHRM, 2013; p. 57), we can only know about the respondents who have gone "above and beyond." It's possible that there may be many other employers in the sample who are also providing adequate and reasonable breastfeeding support according to the law. Nevertheless, the results of the survey are hopeful if the increase in lactation/mother's rooms is an indication of a culture shift that may be difficult to quantify otherwise.

Other areas that were included in the survey are also relevant to breastfeeding in the workplace and offer room for improvement. One survey question concerns the provision of lactation support services, defined as "lactation consulting and education" (SHRM, 2013; p. 34). The results indicate that a disappointing eight percent of respondents offer these services. Finally, only one percent of respondents offer the "family friendly" benefit of bringing children younger than one year old to work on a regular basis. (Incidentally, five percent of respondents allow employees to bring their pets to work). At any rate, the benefit of being able to breastfeed as opposed to pumping in the workplace has a lot to offer breastfeeding mothers and their children, and is discussed briefly below.

Employment Laws and Benefits

Whether the employer is in the educational setting or elsewhere, they will have to comply with federal and state laws regarding provisions for breastfeeding women. The federal ACA that passed in 2010, requires employers to provide "reasonable break time for an employee to express breast milk for her nursing child for one year after the child's birth each time such employee has need to express the milk" (U.S. Department of Labor Wage and Hour Division, n.d.). The Break Time for Nursing Mothers Law applies to employers with greater than 50 employees. According to this law, employers are also obligated to provide "reasonable break time that will vary by employee." Additionally, the federal law applies only to employees who are paid hourly as opposed to salaried. This provision has proven to be challenging for mothers in some settings as discussed previously.

Mothers who live in states without workplace laws and for whom the federal mandate does not apply, may find it very difficult to continue to breastfeed upon return to the workplace following birth. Data suggests that state laws vary widely, not only because they may or may not have a law in place, but also by the individual provisions. The latest report indicates that only 24 states have laws in place regarding the workplace environment (National Conference of State Legislatures, 2011). By way of clarification, the federal law does not supersede state laws. Whichever law provides the most protection to the individual employee, state or federal, stands. The ACA is still relatively new and, generally speaking, many agree that it is exceedingly complex.

Employment benefits are one way for employers to not only meet the requirements of state and federal breastfeeding laws, but to extend policies that benefit all parties—women, children, families, and the employers alike. Family-friendly policies, such as the provision of lactation support, increase employee satisfaction and therefore improve employee retention. Other benefits of lactation programs are decreased medical costs to employers (because of fewer insurance claims), and decreased absenteeism of employees (because children are not sick as often, requiring parents to stay home from work). The full provisions of the ACA are beyond the scope of this book and can be located in any number of sources; however, benefit packages for employees will need to consider other provisions in addition to the Break Time for Nursing Mothers Law discussed above. Expanded preventive services for women under the ACA that employers will need to consider with regard to benefit packages include "breastfeeding supplies and services" (USDHHS, Human Resources Services Administration, n.d.).

Finally, in addition to the aforementioned laws and benefits, other benefits to support breastfeeding would ideally expand on current policies regarding lactation programs to provide mothers with direct access to their babies. Innovative strategies that provide flexibility during the workday to allow mothers to either go to their babies or have their babies brought to them stand to increase breastfeeding duration, lowering excess risk of acute and chronic illness. Examples of policies that may achieve this goal are telecommuting, extended paid leave, and implementing onsite childcare (USDHHS, 2011).

Achieving Breastfeeding Goals for All

As it appears that the trend toward the establishment of a workplace culture that supports breastfeeding is on the rise, employers will likely be faced with greater expectations from employees with regard to policies that support them in their roles at work and at home. Although the above section highlights more general employer considerations, the college and university setting is also an employer, and therefore expected to adhere to federal and state laws. Additionally, the university setting is one employment sector that has received little attention with regard to breastfeeding programs (SHRM, 2013). To highlight the need for university-specific information regarding breastfeeding support, one need only look at some demographic data within the higher education setting.

Whether faculty members, staff, or students, mothers in the higher education setting reasonably constitute a substantial number of women. To start, the total proportion of women faculty compared with men faculty in degree-granting institutions in the U.S. has been on the rise since the mid-1980s, as evidenced by the fact that the total proportion of women faculty in 1987 was 33.2% compared with 48.2% in 2011 (National Center for Education Statistics (NCES), 2011a). This is good news. Unfortunately, women faculty have also struggled to keep pace with men in equal positions due largely to their role as a mother. Therefore, policy recommendations in higher education include paid and unpaid leave for pregnancy, family care, reduced workload, and stopping the tenure clock for up to two years following birth (Vancour, 2009).

Reasonably speaking, not all women faculty members in the higher education setting are of childbearing age. Even those who are of childbearing age may not be choosing to breastfeed following birth. However, in the U.S. in 2010, the total number of women faculty in academia reached nearly 800,000. Beyond faculty on campus, the total number of women students enrolled in a four-year degree-granting institution reached almost 12 million (NCES, 2011b). Nationally, approximately 75% of women giving birth will initiate breastfeeding which suggests that a large number of women returning to the academic setting following birth may be trying to combine breastfeeding with professional or student responsibilities. These data do not include graduate students or other women who may be employed in any number of roles in this setting, such as food service, campus security, administration, and human resources, suggesting an even greater number of women who may be impacted by university breastfeeding programs.

To our knowledge, this book is the first of its kind to highlight unique and specific challenges to the establishment of a breastfeeding support program on a university campus. As alluded to in the Editors' Notes, a university campus is much like a small city. All community members, those with diverse demographics with regard to race and ethnicity, as well as employees who fall under multiple levels of employment categories and varying levels of education, will require the benefit of careful planning and implementation of breastfeeding policies that benefit all. For example, given the health disparities discussed previously among breastfeeding mothers by race, it will be critical to provide programs that are culturally compatible with social norms of varying constituencies. Of note, the editors attempted to include a chapter from a Historically Black College/University (HBCU) without success. This does not mean that programs do not exist among HBCU settings. Programs that are implemented within this setting might assist in the dissemination of important culturally specific considerations for women of African descent on campus.

Finally, it will be critical for those responsible for the planning, oversight, and evaluation to consult diverse stakeholders who can assist with the connections between health and work, and the availability of valuable resources that may assist in guiding program components, such as the Business Case for Breastfeeding (USDHHS, HRSA, n.d.) and the Surgeon General's report (USDHHS, 2011).

References

Abdulwadud, O. A., & Snow, M. E. (2012). Interventions in the workplace to support breastfeeding for women in employment. *Cochrane Database Syst Rev, 10*, CD006177. doi: 10.1002/14651858.CD006177.pub3

American Academy of Pediatrics (APA). (2012). Breastfeeding and the use of human milk. *Pediatrics, 129*(3), e827-841. doi: 10.1542/peds.2011-3552

Bartick, M., & Reinhold, A. (2010). The burden of suboptimal breastfeeding in the United States: A pediatric cost analysis. *Pediatrics, 125*(5), e1048-1056. doi: 10.1542/peds.2009-1616

Centers for Disease Control and Prevention. (2013). Progress in increasing breastfeeding and reducing racial/ethnic differences - United States, 2000-2008 births. *MMWR: Morbidity and Mortality Weekly Report, 62*, 77-80.

Galson, S. K. (2009). The 25th anniversary of the Surgeon General's Workshop on Breastfeeding and Human Lactation: The status of breastfeeding today. *Public Health Reports, 124*(3), 356.

Ip, S., Chung, M., Raman, G., Trikalinos, T. A., & Lau, J. (2009). A summary of the Agency for Healthcare Research and Quality's evidence report on breastfeeding in developed countries. *Breastfeeding Medicine, 4 Suppl 1*, S17-30. doi: 10.1089/bfm.2009.0050

National Center for Educational Statistics (NCES). (2011a). *Number of faculty in degree-granting institutions by employment status, sex, control, and level of institution. Selected years, fall 1970 through fall 2011*. Retrieved on January 20, 2014 from http://nces.ed.gov/programs/digest/d12/tables/dt12_290.asp

National Center for Educational Statistics (NCES). (2011b). *Total fall enrollment in degree-greanting institutions, by attendance status, sex of student and control of institution: Selected years, 1947 through 2011*. Retrieved on January 20, 2014 from http://nces.ed.gov/programs/digest/d12/tables/dt12_221.asp

National Conference of State Legislatures (2011). *State breastfeeding laws*. Retrieved on January 20, 2014 from http://www.ncsl.org/research/health/breastfeeding-state-laws.aspx

Perrine, C. G., Scanlon, K. S., Li, R., Odom, E., & Grummer-Strawn, L. M. (2012). Baby-friendly hospital practices and meeting exclusive breastfeeding intention. *Pediatrics, 130*(1), 54-60. doi: 10.1542/peds.2011-3633

Society for Human Resource Management (SHRM). (2013). Research and Metrics. Survey Findings. *2013 State of Employee Benefits in the Workplace Series.* Retrieved on January 20, 2014 from http://www.shrm.org/research/surveyfindings/articles/documents/13-0245%202013_empbenefits_fnl.pdf

Tuttle, C. R., & Slavit, W. I. (2009). Establishing the business case for breastfeeding. *Breastfeeding Medicine, 4 Suppl 1*, S59-62. doi: 10.1089/bfm.2009.0031

U.S. Department of Health and Human Services (USDHHS), Health Resources Services Administration (HRSA), Maternal Child Health Bureau. (n.d.). *Business case for breastfeeding.* Retrieved on January 19, 2014 from http://mchb.hrsa.gov/pregnancyandbeyond/breastfeeding/

U.S. Department of Health and Human Services (USDHHS). (n.d.). *Healthy People 2020. Topics and objectives, maternal, infant and child health.* MICH 21-22. Retrieved on January 20, 2014 from http://www.healthypeople.gov/2020/topicsobjectives2020/objectiveslist.aspx?topicId=26

U.S. Department of Health and Human Services (USDHHS). (2011). *The surgeon general's call to action to support breastfeeding.* Rockville MD.

U.S. Department of Health and Human Services (USDHHS), Human Resources and Services Administration (HRSA). (n.d.). Women's Preventive Services Guidelines. *Breastfeeding support, supplies and counseling.* Retrieved on January 20, 2014 from http://www.hrsa.gov/womensguidelines/

U.S. Department of Labor, Bureau of Labor Statistics. (2009). *The Editor's Desk,* Labor force participation of mothers with infants in 2008. Retrieved on January 7, 2014 from http://www.bls.gov/opub/ted/2009/may/wk4/art04.htm

U.S. Department of Labor, Wage and Hour Division. (n.d.). *Fact sheet break time for nursing mothers under FLSA.* Retrieved on January 19, 2014 from http://www.dol.gov/whd/regs/compliance/whdfs73.htm

Vancour, M.L. (2009). Motherhood, balance, and health behaviours of academic women. *Journal of the Motherhood Initiative for Research and Community Involvement, 11*(1).

Weimer, Jon P. (2001). *The economic benefits of breastfeeding: A review and analysis.* United States Department of Agriculture, Economic Research Service.

Chapter Two
GW, A Breastfeeding-Friendly University

Erica Hayton

The George Washington University (GW) is a private university founded in 1812 by an Act of Congress. There are approximately 10,000 undergraduates and 14,000 graduate students across all of our locations, plus an additional 1,000 non-degree students. The University employs approximately 11,000 faculty and staff, of which 5,500 are in regular, benefits-eligible positions. Benefits are extended to all regular full-time and part-time faculty and staff who work a minimum of 14 hours a week.

GW has three campuses, the largest of which is Foggy Bottom Campus, which sits just four blocks from the White House in the heart of Washington, D.C. The 42 acres of our Foggy Bottom campus include a metro stop, more than 100 campus buildings, and a wide variety of shops and restaurants. Countless numbers of visitors come to or pass through our campus annually. The Mount Vernon Campus, the smallest of our campuses, sits fewer than three miles from our Foggy Bottom campus and a mile northwest of Georgetown University in Washington, D.C. Despite the close proximity to Foggy Bottom, the Mount Vernon campus feels much more like a small liberal arts college. The campus is home to many of our freshman and some sophomores, as well as our Honors Program, Women's Leadership Program, Interior Design Program, University Writing Program, Department of Forensic Science, and GW Pre-College Summer Program for high school students. The Virginia Science and Technology Campus, the fastest growing of our campuses, is located approximately 25 miles northwest of Foggy Bottom in the middle of Northern Virginia's technology corridor. Once a rural landscape, these days it seems like new businesses and housing developments pop up daily in this area. We have five buildings spread out on 100 acres of land. Two buildings are primarily intended for administrative purposes, with most of the Information Technology and Finance groups on this campus, as well as half of the Human Resources division, and a number of other administrative offices. The other three buildings are used for academics and research, including 20 graduate degree programs, the National Crash Analysis Center, and collaborations with the National Science Foundation, government, and industry.

The Vision for a Breastfeeding Friendly University

Work-life programs have been around for at least eight years at the George Washington University, but it wasn't until mid-September 2011 that a true focus on breastfeeding support took shape. It was during a small breakfast meeting at the house of our university President, led by the wife of our new Provost, that the idea for GW's Breastfeeding Friendly University Project (BFUP) took shape. Our Provost's wife, an International Board Certified Lactation Consultant, described a recent session she attended on the topic of becoming a Baby Friendly Hospital at the International Lactation Consultants Association (ILCA) conference. Already familiar with the specifics of this designation, her mind began to wonder as she pondered what a Baby Friendly University would look like. As she described to the group that September morning, she had a vision of GW becoming the model for university-based breastfeeding support and was looking for others to join her in making this initiative a reality.

From a relatively small group of breakfast guests has grown an initiative with more than 100 members on the mailing list and a number of subcommittees. It would be difficult to list all of the members of the BFUP, but some notable and more active members include the following (by title only):

- Dean, School of Public Health
- Dean, School of Nursing
- Vice Provost, Diversity and Inclusion
- Senior Associate Dean, School of Nursing
- Chair and Professor, Environmental and Occupational Health
- Professor, Obstetrics and Gynecology
- Assistant Professor, Anthropology
- Human Resources (HR) Director, Benefits and Wellness
- Executive Director, University Events
- Director, Midwife Program, GW University Hospital
- Clinical Manager, GW University Hospital Childbirth Center
- RNs (multiple members), GW University Hospital

Full committee meetings are held two to three times per semester. However, members of the committee meet with much more frequency within subcommittees to move forward specific focus areas or to work on defined objectives. Additionally, in spring 2013 a steering committee was formed to help provide further direction for the project. The steering committee meets monthly.

While there are various plans underway directly or indirectly related to this project, the key areas of focus for the Breastfeeding Friendly University Project initially included:

- Community Support (both our own GW community and the larger D.C. community),

- Hospital Partnership,

- Professional Education

In summer 2012, the BFUP was provided a dedicated space through GW's School of Public Health and Health Services for offering group meetings, educational sessions, and one-on-one consultations. The room also allows space for a lending library for mothers and professionals and for potential future equipment rentals. It should not be ignored, however, that members of the BFUP committee spent many months writing emails and proposals, and meeting with various GW leaders to advocate for a dedicated meeting space prior to receiving it.

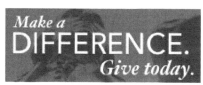

Figure 2.1 GW Give Today

An important note in discussing our current and future programming is that to date no University funding has been allocated specifically for this project. We initially had a small budget provided directly from donors, which we used for equipment for our BFUP room and to host an event in October 2012 to formally announce the project to the GW and D.C. community. We have worked with our Development Office on fundraising opportunities and have a dedicated website for the project (breastfeeding.gwu.edu) that includes a "Give Today" button for people to contribute to the project (Figure 2.1). Additional funding has primarily come from the Human Resources' existing budget under work-life and wellness programming. It is likely in the next year, as the project continues to grow, that we will need to either be more aggressive in our fundraising efforts, seek outside grants to support specific programs, or request funding directly from the University.

As described during our event in October 2012, the video of which is available on the breastfeeding.gwu.edu website, we see the Breastfeeding Friendly University Project in three stages. The first stage, which began when the Project was initially launched in 2011 and continued into fall 2012, was our formation stage (Figure 2.2). While we were able to make a good deal of progress in terms of what we offer to breastfeeding mothers during this time, it was mainly focused on building support for the Project, creating an inventory of our current programs and resources, and researching best practices in lactation

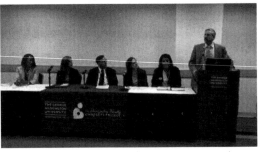

Figure 2.2 GW Breastfeeding Group Photo

support. The second or needs assessment stage, which kicked off following the October 2012 event, is focused on collecting feedback from our community about what's most needed in terms of breastfeeding support and determining what is realistic for our institution and our partners to achieve. The third stage, or implementation stage, is when we expect to introduce major changes, particularly those that require additional support and/or funding. These could include anything from lactation counseling services, to paid parental leave, to a dedicated parent support center — all dependent on our needs assessment findings and the level of support received.

> BEST PRACTICE: Soliciting feedback from the community on GW's lactation program facilitated their planning process.

Community Support

Community support means a number of things for the Breastfeeding Friendly University Project. First and foremost, it focuses on how we better support our own faculty, staff, and students. This may be in terms of infrastructure, policies, programs, or resources that allow a new mother to continue breastfeeding, even after returning to work or class. Beyond our immediate community, it also looks at how GW serves our larger Foggy Bottom and D.C. community. It may be that some of the programs and resources we offer in our own GW community can also be more broadly provided. It considers what role GW has in the larger discussion about breastfeeding and work-life balance. It also looks at fostering valuable partnerships with other groups and organizations in the community who are working towards a common goal.

Hospital Partnership

The George Washington University Hospital, despite the name, is a privately held hospital that operates separately from the University. However, it is on our campus, shares our name, is a place of work for many of our faculty and residents, and is where many of our GW community choose to give birth. As such, we felt that it was critical to partner with the hospital to ensure that they share in our commitment to support breastfeeding mothers and their partners. We believe that we are responsible for preparing our leaders of tomorrow, as well as our faculty and staff, and to make a larger impact on society.

Professional Education

One of the unique aspects of a university as compared to other organizations is that we don't just have employees, we also have students. In particular, we have medical students, nursing students, and public health students, all of whom are being given the skills needed to promote health for their future patients or clients. A university is a perfect platform for training these future practitioners, not only in the benefits of breastfeeding, but in the nuts and bolts of how to support a new mother who is first learning to breastfeed or struggling with a breastfeeding challenge. We want to not only affect breastfeeding within our GW community, but also to prepare future healthcare providers to promote breastfeeding in their own communities.

Supporting our Breastfeeding Mothers

Starting from almost nothing, the first thing those working on the Community Support subcommittee sought to do was better understand what other organizations offered in order to define current best practices, as well as ways we might further raise the bar. One specific tool we found particularly helpful was the criteria for the D.C. and Maryland Breastfeeding Coalitions Breastfeeding Friendly Workplace Award. Our thought was that if this is the criteria used to determine a "Breastfeeding Friendly Workplace," it would be a good guide for identifying where we needed to start. The award includes an extensive list of criteria, divided up between Bronze, Silver, and Gold, and categorized by support, time, education, and space. Support includes breastfeeding policies, education/training, and opportunities for mom-to-mom support. Time looks at unpaid/paid leave, flexible work arrangements, and on-site childcare. Education includes resources, classes, a lending library, and opportunities for one-on-one consultation. Place speaks to all of the details of private space and furnishings for pumping and breastfeeding.

The Community Support subcommittee looked at each of the criteria to determine which we already had in place, which we could easily accomplish within the next year, and which would be more challenging to accomplish, primarily due to resource limitations. We started this review shortly after the launch of the Breastfeeding Friendly Project in 2011 and quickly worked to check as many of these items off the list as possible through new programs and resources. It was with great pride that within one year's time we were able to make enough forward movement to be selected as a recipient for an award in 2012. We were the only university on the 2012 award recipient list.

> BEST PRACTICE: Framing their approach toward best practices, GW used the criteria from state breastfeeding coalitions' Breastfeeding Friendly Workplace Award as a starting point.

Establishing Well-Conceived and Received Motherhood Rooms

When the Breastfeeding Friendly University Project first launched in fall 2011, we had only one dedicated "Motherhood Room," our name for lactation rooms, across all three of our campuses, and it was on our Virginia Science and Technology Campus in Ashburn, VA. When mothers contacted HR in need of a Motherhood Room on the Foggy Bottom campus, we generally set them up in a HR meeting room or a spare office. On our Mount Vernon Campus, we had two swing spaces, one of which was the library conference room.

Like many urban institutions, space on our Foggy Bottom campus is considered a precious resource; the demand far outweighs the supply (Figure 2.3). In addition, real estate costs in D.C. are near the top of the national rankings, and given the location of our Foggy Bottom Campus in particular, leases come at a premium. So we knew that trying to advocate for dedicated Motherhood Rooms was going to be an uphill battle. In fact, it is one that was started long before the Breastfeeding Friendly University Project kick-off and took at least

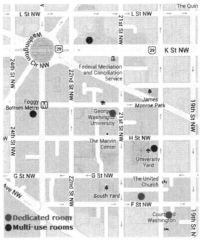

Figure 2.3 GW Map

two to three years to make real gains. Our first room, one of only three dedicated rooms currently on the Foggy Bottom campus, is the size of a changing room and was constructed by adding walls to a corner which was previously open space. It is truly an example of creative problem solving. Despite its small size, it's large enough to fit a comfortable chair and small table. It is centrally located on campus, sitting on the second floor of our community center, and is right next to the women's restroom. Scheduling is officially done by requesting access to a Google Calendar through our Faculty and Staff Service Center, but because the room is not locked except when occupied (it has a vacant/occupied lock on it), it is often used as needed without being scheduled. We have many times debated whether it would be better to more strictly enforce a scheduling requirement, or to provide for the flexibility currently available with an unlocked space. However, since we do not have a staff member on-site to help manage the space, it would be difficult for us to do anything other than the status quo from a practical standpoint. The downside, of course, is that someone could schedule the space only to find that it is already in use by a drop-in. A middle ground would be to use either a keypad lock or card entry system and limit access to those who request it through the Faculty and Staff Service Center. Unfortunately, both those options come at a cost beyond which we were able to fund given our previously mentioned budget constraints.

> BEST PRACTICE: GW leveraged resources to support efforts, particularly given a limited budget. The creative use of Google Calendar for scheduling purposes is one example of this approach.

From that first dedicated room on our Foggy Bottom campus, we have continued to grow. While we would love to have a Motherhood Room in every building on campus, we recognize the realities of space availability. Instead, we agreed on a goal to identify either a dedicated or shared room within a five-minute walk from any building. The benefit of an urban campus is that most of our buildings on the Foggy Bottom and Mount Vernon campuses fit into a relatively small space, so we can cover the five-minute walking rule with three to four strategically located rooms on Foggy Bottom and just one room on Mount Vernon. Our Virginia Science and Technology Campus is another story. Though we only have four buildings, each is more than a five-minute walk from the next, and there is not a consistent pedestrian path between all of the buildings. We knew immediately that for this campus, the ideal would be a room in each building.

Space, particularly on an urban campus, is at a premium. To be successful in our efforts, we needed to acknowledge that we were one of many looking for space and set our sights on what was reasonable. Though we have yet to meet our goal, we are not far off the mark. After receiving our first dedicated room on the Foggy Bottom campus, we successfully negotiated for a second space near the southern edge of our campus. The room was a former storage closet that required some painting, but otherwise proved to be a nice size and well located. In May 2013 we opened our third dedicated room as part of the renovation of our Support Building, which is the home base for most of our housekeeping and grounds workers. Through our discussions with colleagues across campus, we also learned of two multi-use spaces that could be used for Motherhood Rooms and had served this purpose as needed in the past. While each is limited in access, one to law school faculty, staff, and students, and the other to those in our schools of medicine, nursing, and public health, the location of each room fills an important geographic gap. Those who would most likely wish to use either of these two rooms also likely fulfill the access requirements. Finally, our dedicated BFUP room, located on K Street, provides a convenient location for some of our off-campus departments.

The one area of campus currently not covered under our five-minute ideal, though it is not actually on campus at all, are the offices we have in leased space down 21st Street. We hope to identify a space along this corridor in the near future, though this will also become less and less of an issue as we continue to reduce our use of leased space in favor of moving departments from Foggy Bottom to our Virginia Science and Technology Campus, and increasing our use of telecommuting and hoteling space as an alternative to assigned work space.

Beyond our Foggy Bottom campus, we were able to secure a dedicated space on our Mount Vernon Campus that is almost exactly in the middle of campus, making it a five-minute walk from all other buildings. We also have dedicated spaces in three of the four buildings on the Virginia Science and Technology Campus. The one building that does not currently have a Motherhood Room is primarily an academic and research building in which most, if not all, of the faculty and staff have their own offices. While we will continue to advocate for a dedicated space in this building, particularly for students and visitors, we believe the need for a dedicated space in this building is limited. We also hope to continue to add to our network of multiuse spaces to provide more options on all of our campuses.

Similar to our original dedicated room on the Foggy Bottom campus, all of our dedicated rooms have vacant/occupied locks, but are otherwise available on a first-come, first-serve basis. This has not proven to be an issue thus far, but may be something we need to reconsider if scheduling conflicts arise.

The next step after securing dedicated space is determining furnishings and accessories for each room. To provide consistency across all of our dedicated rooms, we developed a Motherhood Room furnishings list that would serve as a minimum requirement for each space. The list includes the following:

- Comfortable chair
- Table
- Power outlet
- Vacant/Occupied lock

- Bulletin board
- Clock
- Trash can
- Extension cord
- Art print and frame
- Parenting magazines (currently *Parents* and *Working Mother*)
- Memo pad, pens and push pins (for leaving "Milk Memos" on the bulletin board)
- White noise machines (as available – repurposed from HR)

We have been fortunate thus far that all of the chairs and tables have come from our university furniture inventory, where we collect furniture no longer needed after a renovation or redesign. The white noise machines we only added to the list because we had a number of them in our HR inventory, though they are a nice addition when a room is in a more public space with thin walls. Some of our mothers have expressed discomfort at knowing others could hear their pumps in action. Many of the other items we tried, when possible, to repurpose from our HR inventory. Our HR team has made a number of moves over the last five years, so it is not unusual for us to have unneeded bulletin boards, trash cans, etc. sitting in storage. The remaining items we have bought out of our HR budget. For the art print, we selected Maternity by Pablo Picasso, which can be purchased online for a relatively low cost. We were also able to find affordable wood frames online to match the colors in the print. Additionally, subscriptions for both *Parents* and *Working Mother* magazines are available for a very low annual or multi-year subscription cost.

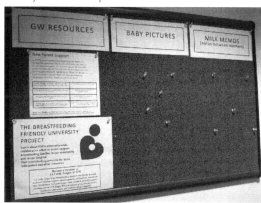

One furnishing that we focused a little more attention on was the bulletin board included in each room (Figure 2.4). Rather than put up just a plain bulletin board, one of the student-staff members from our work-life team in HR developed a standard template we use on each of the

Figure 2.4 GW Breastfeeding Bulletin Board

boards. It divides the board into three sections: one third for information on programs and resources available to faculty and staff related to breastfeeding or parenting, one third for space where mothers can hang pictures of their babies, and one third for mothers to write "Milk Memos" or notes to one another. We don't know yet how well utilized the space for pictures and memos will be, but based on our research and discussions with other organizations that have strong lactation programs, we learned that building a sense of community among breastfeeding mothers can be valuable to those using the spaces and make the rooms feel less sterile.

> BEST PRACTICE: At GW, breastfeeding support is about more than just providing programs and resources. It is about building a sense of community with and among parents.

Our Motherhood Rooms do not currently have multi-user pumps, as many other organizations offer. However, we recently entered into a partnership with Hygeia that includes Hygeia providing us a number of free hospital grade, multi-user pumps, as well as discounts on additional pumps. Our community members also receive discounts to buy accessory sets for these shared pumps, as well as for their own electric or manual pumps. Prior to partnering with Hygeia, we had a number of meetings with another vendor who was equally interested in a partnership with GW; however, we did not feel like they were a good fit for GW or the Breastfeeding Friendly University Project at the time. We chose to work with Hygeia because they produced the first eco-friendly pump, fitting with our GW value of sustainability, and they are one of the very few World Health Organization (WHO) Code compliant pump companies. Our plans are to have a multi-use pump in each of our dedicated rooms in the near future.

> BEST PRACTICE: GW was selective in their partnerships—only choosing those that truly aligned with their vision, like Hygeia with their eco-friendly pump and WHO Code compliance.

Creating a Breastfeeding Policy for GW Working Moms

In fall 2013, after nearly a year of work with our general counsel's office and key stakeholders, we finalized a formal Breastfeeding Policy for GW. The policy speaks to a nursing mother's rights under the law, including her right to breastfeed wherever she and her child are allowed to be, her right to reasonable lactation breaks, and her right to be provided a non-bathroom space, shielded from view and free from intrusion of co-workers and the public. It also details some of the resources available to nursing mothers through the University with links for more information. Finally, it provides guidance to mothers who feel they were denied an appropriate accommodation or who have been discriminated against or harassed as a nursing mother.

We are finalizing with our legal counsel a Children in the Workplace policy. While the policy does not directly speak to breastfeeding, it provides further guidance on when it is or is not appropriate for a child to be in the workplace. This is important because the draft breastfeeding policy states that a woman "may breastfeed her infant in any public or private location on campus where the mother and child are authorized to be." The Children in the Workplace policy will further define that authorized space. While this policy was initially drafted prior to the highly publicized event at a neighboring university where a faculty member brought her sick baby into the classroom and breastfed while lecturing, the media response to this event further emphasized the importance of both policies and how they fit together. This event made headlines locally, but it largely focused on whether or not it was appropriate for the faculty member to breastfeed in class, rather than whether it was appropriate to bring a sick child into the workplace and potentially expose many more people. Our Children in the Workplace policy will restrict sick children from the workplace to protect the health of our community. It also protects children from accessing hazardous locations. It allows managers flexibility in permitting children into non-hazardous work areas and emphasizes our back-up care and other work-life benefits available to parents needing alternate care arrangements. The goal of our two policies is to support a woman's right to breastfeed, but also to recognize the boundaries of a work environment.

A final policy that we have had in place since 2005, but will likely become more important as the Breastfeeding Friendly University Project moves forward, is our Flexible Work Arrangements policy, which includes telecommuting, compressed work week(s), and other flexible scheduling options. By providing flexible work options to our breastfeeding mothers, we may make it easier to find time to breastfeed or pump during or around work hours, or perhaps for the woman to breastfeed/pump in the comfort of her own home. It is well known that D.C. has one of the worst average commutes nationwide, and often our employees do not live close to campus due to the previously mentioned high real estate costs. If telecommuting and other flexible work arrangements allow our working mothers to spend less time in rush hour commutes, that's more potential time spent with their babies. Moving forward we hope to work more directly with new and expecting mothers to help them understand their flexible work arrangement options and how to make a business case to their supervisor to approve such arrangements.

> BEST PRACTICE: As part of GW's Innovative Task Force, the University made a commitment to provide telecommuting, in part as a space reduction measure, but more importantly as a way to promote and support employees' work-life balance.

Revisiting Time Off and Leave to Support Healthy Families

Based on research that we have done as part of the Breastfeeding Friendly University Project, we know that no amount of workplace support can compare to giving a mother more time at home with her baby. We provide GW-paid short-term disability coverage for full-time faculty and staff beginning at two years of service (though amount of coverage varies for staff between two and five years). Our current coverage allows for an average of four weeks income replacement after a vaginal birth and six weeks after a Cesarean birth, assuming no additional complications.

Additionally, we recently updated our sick time-off policy to allow sick time to be used for all Family Medical Leave Act (FMLA) covered leaves. Based on our benchmarking of peer institutions, this is a fairly unique provision. Previously, our sick time policy could only be used either during the medical recovery period for the mother after birth (what is not covered by short-term disability) or if her child was sick, since sick leave can be used to care for a sick family member. However, the "bonding" period after the mother had recovered from birth, but still wished to be at home with her child was not covered by sick time. This change to the policy allows for coverage during the bonding period, as well as coverage for partners on FMLA approved leave. In addition to the FMLA, GW also is required to comply with the D.C. Family and Medical Leave Act, which extends the 12 weeks under the Federal Act to 16 weeks for both the individual's own health condition, as well as care of a family member. So, under a vaginal birth with no complications, which generally has a six-week recovery period, it is likely that an employee would be approved for up to 22 weeks of leave under D.C. FMLA. Like many universities, we provide 12 days a year of paid sick time off and allow employees to accrue up to a maximum of 180 days of sick time. For a woman who has worked at GW for a number of years and has not used a substantial number of her sick days previously, between sick time and GW-paid short-term disability, she may be able to stay home for a significant period of time, while still receiving a regular paycheck.

BEST PRACTICE: GW's new leave policy specifically supports "bonding" and is a unique provision among benchmarked universities.

Beginning January 2014, GW is going one step further by introducing a new paid parental leave policy as part of a "family-friendly" benefits strategy. Under this new leave benefit, regular full-time staff, with two years or more of benefit-eligible service, will receive six weeks of paid leave immediately following the birth or adoption of a child. This benefit will run concurrent with short-term disability for the birth mother. Following the six weeks of paid leave, employees will still be eligible to use accrued sick or annual time for the remainder of the FMLA-approved leave period. Faculty are already eligible for Parental

Childcare Leave under GW's Faculty Code, providing release from teaching responsibilities and service responsibilities for one semester, with full salary and benefits, following birth or adoption of a child.

Healthy Pregnancy Program to Promote Positive Health Outcomes

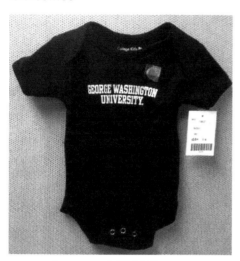

Figure 2.5 GW Onesie

In 2012, we introduced the GW Healthy Pregnancy Program in partnership with United Healthcare (UHC). The program is open to faculty, staff, and their family members on our medical plan. The core of the program is telephonic case management by experienced nurses through UHC. There is an initial assessment in which we prepare those signing up for the program that they will be asked a number of personal medical questions necessary to assess any pregnancy risks. Based on the outcome of that assessment and future discussions, the regularity of the phone calls between participant and nurse are determined. Participating women also have 24/7 access to a special nurse line, as well as educational materials provided by UHC. In 2012 the incentive for participating in the program was a GW infant onesie (Figure 2.5). In 2013, we were able to make the business case during our internal benefits renewal process for up to $250 in incentives paid through payroll. Under our 2013 incentive strategy, mothers who enroll during the first trimester are eligible for a $100 payment. If a mother waits until her second trimester to enroll, she receives $75. Regardless of enrollment period, any mother who completes the program is eligible for an additional $150 payment.

Aside from the medical benefit of this program, both in terms of the individual and the financial impact to our self-insured institution, it provides us with a target audience for breastfeeding resources and support. Using MailChimp, an online system for designing and sending email marketing campaigns, we have developed an automated monthly email newsletter for our Healthy Pregnancy participants, timed to their due date. The newsletter allows us the opportunity to feature many of our work-life benefits, including our Employee Assistance Program, Work-Life Resource and Referral services, Health Advocacy, and classes available through our GW Hospital. We have also developed a special breastfeeding newsletter for those who expressed an interest in this topic as part of their Healthy Pregnancy program registration.

BEST PRACTICE: Identifying ways to utilize technologies, like MailChimp, to support lactation programs provides innovative methods for promoting breastfeeding, lactation services, and other topics.

In addition to regular communications and a webpage specific to Healthy Pregnancy that includes a number of breastfeeding resources, after we receive word of a birth, we send a packet home to the family with a GW infant onesie (still provided despite the new incentive) and additional resources, including a flyer for our La Leche League meetings. We also recently signed a contract with one of our work-life vendors to offer a special ParentGuidance program beginning September 1, 2013, which provides specialized outbound telephonic support services to respond to parenting needs and concerns, as well as a "New Baby Kit" mailed to the participant's home. The program also includes support to help prepare participants for their return to work.

Bringing Support Options to GW

One of our best on-site support programs currently available to all of our GW and D.C. community members is our monthly La Leche League meetings. These are provided by our Project lead, who is an IBCLC. We have two meeting times, each held monthly. The daytime meeting is held the third Tuesday of every month from 12:00-1:30 p.m. to accommodate participants' lunch schedules. The second, more recently added, is our evening meeting held the first Tuesday of every month from 5:30-7:00 p.m. for the after-work crowd. The meetings are held in our BFUP dedicated meeting space, which allows not only enough room for our mothers to meet, but access to our lending library and other resources. While participants are encouraged to join the La Leche League of Maryland, Delaware, and the District of Columbia to support the GW group for an annual donation of $25, the meetings are free and open to the public. We have 50 mothers who are currently or have been members of GW's La Leche League since it began in late 2011, as well as four leaders in training who hope to go on to lead additional meetings either at GW or elsewhere. To date, the La Leche League participants have been a good mix of GW employees and members from the larger community. Admittedly, if not for the passion of our Project lead and willingness to donate her time for these meetings, it would be very difficult for us to offer them.

BEST PRACTICE: GW expands its lactation services with an open invitation for community members to join their on-site monthly La Leche League meetings led by their Project Lead.

Meetings held once per month, while standard for La Leche League, may not be enough for nursing mothers. We are, therefore, working on establishing weekly meetings for mothers to simply get together and support one another. Ideally, we would like to have a daily opportunity for a nursing mother to get support. One way we are working to build this capacity is by establishing a partnership with our School of Public Health and Health Services, School of Medicine and School of Nursing to create a training program that would certify students as lactation support providers. This would then allow us to set up regular office hours staffed by these certified individuals to meet with nursing mothers one-on-one. Such a program would not only benefit our community members, but would be another skill our students could include on their resume.

> BEST PRACTICE: By including students in this project and training them to be lactation support providers, GW not only increases the number of individuals supporting their efforts, but also provides a valuable learning opportunity those students can take with them to future careers.

In addition to direct breastfeeding support, we are looking at hosting regular information sessions for expecting GW mothers and partners to discuss GW's benefits and programs in detail. This session would include an overview of our various leave programs, how they work together, and how to complete the process to request coverage under each program. It would include a discussion of our many work-life benefits, including our childcare referral service, back-up care, on-site childcare, health advocacy, and our employee assistance program. It might also include some down-to-earth feedback from mothers about what to expect after the birth of their children and tips on finding work-life balance in the new world of parenthood. These sessions could be offered both in person in our meeting space, as well as virtually, for relatively no cost aside from the HR staff time required to develop the program and then provide it. In the spirit of university collaboration, we are currently working with Johns Hopkins University to model our information sessions after their successful Baby Shower program.

We are looking at how we can better partner with other organizations to provide further breastfeeding support. Our GW Hospital currently offers breastfeeding classes, as well as birth preparation classes, through a contract with Momease, a local provider of classes, services, and educational tools related to pregnancy. Not only are we working with the hospital to better promote their classes, but we are talking with Momease directly about providing additional classes on campus, as well as potentially subsidizing the costs of these classes for our GW community. The Breastfeeding Center for Greater Washington, adjacent to our Foggy Bottom campus, offers free and low-cost breastfeeding classes, one-on-one lactation consultations, and a fully stocked breastfeeding boutique. They serve as a resource currently for many of our GW breastfeeding moms, and we are looking at potential partnerships with them in the future as well.

Strengthening GW's Breastfeeding Partnerships

We are fortunate at GW to be able to provide a number of work-life benefits to our faculty and staff. As part of the Breastfeeding Friendly University Project, we have reached out to each of our work-life vendors to identify how they can help support our efforts. Our work-life resource and referral service provides referrals for lactation consultants and breastfeeding classes, educational resources on breastfeeding, and a free prenatal kit. Our health advocacy provider also provides support connecting our employees with lactation consultants, as well as assistance with explaining coverage under our medical plans and dealing with medical billing issues. Our Employee Assistance Program has provided us with marketing materials targeted specifically at new parents that we include in our Healthy Pregnancy packet. Finally, our on-site child-care center encourages GW parents to come by the center to breastfeed their babies and provides the space to do so, as does our back-up care provider, who also has a center on GW's campus.

With added coverage required under the Women's Preventive Services provision of the Affordable Care Act, we have worked closely with United Healthcare and our benefits consultants to understand the expanded coverage for lactation support services and pumps. UHC has provided us with a number of informational flyers that we have been able to either directly provide to our employees, or use to develop GW-specific communications.

GW Partners are a Priority, Too

While we do not have any specific programs or resources we can highlight at this time related to partner support, it is important to note that we have not lost sight of the importance of partners in providing breastfeeding support. This may be as simple as providing breastfeeding classes or consultations that are open to both the mother and her partner, or as complex as training programs targeted specifically at the partner and his or her role in supporting the nursing mom. We also think about the role of the partner as we are looking at our policies and benefits. If we can make it easier for a partner to stay home longer with mother and baby, or be able to work a flexible work arrangement and avoid lost time in rush hour commutes, his or her additional time at home may make it that much easier for the mother to breastfeed longer.

Working with Our Neighbors

Since the inception of this project, much work has been done between the GW Hospital and the Breastfeeding Friendly University

Project to better align the Hospital with the goals of the project. A number of hospital staff serve on the Hospital Partnership subcommittee, as well as midwives from the GW Medical Faculty Associates, who solely provide hospital births at the GW Hospital. The subcommittee has successfully advocated for the hiring of additional lactation consultants in the hospital that now provide seven-day-a-week consultation for patients, as well as a serious look at re-organizing the Women's Center to encourage rooming in for mother and baby. The hßospital now has a dedicated lactation room available for both patients and staff. Long term, we hope that through strong advocacy, both within the hospital and from the University community, GW Hospital will complete all ten steps necessary to earn the "Baby Friendly" designation as outlined by the World Health Organization and UNICEF. However, we recognize that this requires a lot of financial, administrative, and personnel resources to achieve and, therefore, will take time.

> BEST PRACTICE: Creating a strong partnership with neighboring maternity hospitals can foster collaborative assistance toward goals for both the hospital and the university (steps 3 and 10 of the Ten Steps to Successful Breastfeeding – see Appendix.)

Educating our Future Practitioners

Our Professional Education work looks at not only what we provide in our own community, but the students we graduate who go on to serve other communities. As part of the Breastfeeding Friendly University Project, we have collaborated with the School of Medicine to include a breastfeeding lecture into the course curriculum for all third-year medical students, as well as a standardized patient experience in which medical students have to individually respond to a patient struggling with a breastfeeding challenge. We are looking to establish similar requirements for the School of Nursing. We are also working closely with our School of Public Health and Health Services to develop the previously mentioned certificate program, as well as a number of research projects to help further inform our project objectives.

Summary

Within a relatively short period of time, GW and the Breastfeeding Friendly Project have made great strides in promoting breastfeeding and better supporting our lactating mothers. Yet there is much to be done. We have only begun to scratch the surface of what is possible at a university, from benefits and policies to research and activism. As the project continues, we are also beginning to take a step back and recognize that breastfeeding support is only one important element in a larger goal of being a family-friendly employer. We want to do our part as an institution to support the children and their parents of our GW community from preconception to adulthood, so they will grow into strong leaders and continue to push the work-life agenda for future generations.

Chapter Three
Breastfeeding Unveiled: Legitimizing Lactation Support as a Workplace Priority at URI

Barb Silver

Before Lactation, the Birth of a University Work-Life Committee

Chartered in 1888 as the state's agricultural school, the University of Rhode Island (URI) is the state's Land, Sea, and Urban Grant public institution. It is located on four campuses across the state. The main campus is in Kingston, in a moderately rural part of Rhode Island, and is home to most of the 12,000 undergraduate students, 4,000 graduate students, 700 tenure-line faculty, and 1,800 staff. The Narragansett Bay campus, home to the highly regarded Graduate School of Oceanography and many research faculty, the urban Providence campus, which offers continuing education and serves predominantly commuter and adult students, and the W. Alton Jones environmental research and conference center campus comprise the other three campuses.

In 2002, the President's Commission on the Status of Women (PCOSW) was formed on the Kingston campus, and out of this commission, a work-life subcommittee was created. In partnership with the ADVANCE grant team described below, this subcommittee became URI's Work-Life Committee (WLC) in 2003, and lactation support became one of its priorities. Founded and co-chaired by Barbara Silver, Assistant Research Professor, Psychology, and Helen Mederer, Professor of Sociology, the WLC is comprised of a volunteer group of 10-15 faculty, staff, and students, and is currently the driving force for essentially all work-life efforts at the University. Silver and Mederer, both social scientists, focus their research and scholarship on work-life and workplace issues, and their outreach on institutional and statewide work-life initiatives.

The WLC is guided by strong philosophical and theoretical frameworks that are grounded in social science research. It envisions work-life supports and workplace flexibility initiatives not as a reflection of outdated cultural expectations, but as a means to bring about the social changes necessary to meet the needs of a diverse 21st-century workforce. Among the guiding principles that inform its efforts, two are most relevant here, and summarize the larger point that lactation support is not a woman's issue, but a societal one that must be openly embraced:

Our work recognizes that the economy depends on families to perform essential unpaid work: to bear and raise the next generation of workers and to support and nurture present and past workers. Workplaces can no longer base policies and practices on the assumption that employers have no responsibility for supporting workers' lives off the job. Work and family are inextricably interconnected, and one cannot function without the other. Research evidence is clear on three points: children are well served when they are cared for in families with shared nurturance responsibility; fathers want to be more involved in family life, but feel constrained by work expectations; and when families make gendered choices about family care, women are much less likely to succeed in even the most family-friendly work environment. Thus, our initiatives are designed to help families make non-gendered choices about work and family life.

Building Lactation Support, One Grant at a Time

It is well known that academic women in science, technology, engineering, and math (STEM) face particular challenges as they compete in male-dominated, highly demanding work arenas, often while simultaneously juggling significant care-giving responsibilities (Ginther, 2006). The STEM disciplines have long been white male bastions, characterized by workers who devote up to 60-80 hours a week to their careers with few family encumbrances. All too often, women proceed more slowly or drop out altogether from the tenure track, in part because of overwhelming workloads combined with care-giving responsibilities. URI was successful in securing two grants to promote the careers of women in STEM, both of which laid the foundation for its current lactation program.

Grant 1: A Major ADVANCEment for URI Women

In 2003, URI was awarded a $3.5 million National Science Foundation ADVANCE Institutional Transformation award. The grant was directed by Barbara Silver and supported by a strong leadership team of senior faculty and administrators. In addition to a unique recruitment program, the grant included an array of retention strategies, many of which were directed toward providing work-life supports.

In 2006, ADVANCE submitted a proposal to the URI Administration for the creation of a prototype lactation room within the space of the ADVANCE office. It was emphasized that this space was a first step only, and that future sites across campus would be identified. The proposal asked for funding to reconfigure the room and presented the following set of rationales:

- The increase in numbers of breastfeeding workers, nationally and at URI;

- Wide-ranging, documented benefits of breastfeeding;

- Legislation, both nationally and in Rhode Island, which at the time was one of 38 states to have a breastfeeding-in-the-workplace law;

- An emphasis that, beyond equity for all breastfeeding women, students, staff, and faculty, this is a workplace, societal, and health issue that impacts everyone;

- A description of the lactation room and how it would be managed;

- An emphasis that the University should assume responsibility for the designation and oversight of future sites on campus.

The proposal section of the grant, with reference to the specific institutional request, was based on best practices in use at progressive institutions that were early leaders in this arena. As well, the ADVANCE team was interested in close monitoring, data collection, and program evaluation, since documented evidenced-based best practices could provide useful background data for other institutions to begin their own programs and for URI to expand our program to other campus sites. Finally, in alignment with the goals of the WLC, we were interested in showcasing this prototype site as a visible and attractive support service to normalize and validate the needs of breastfeeding workers. It was worded as follows:

The ADVANCE program and the President's Commission on the Status of Women are developing a proposal for the identification of several lactation sites on campus, depending on the identified need. We propose that the first site be a small room in the ADVANCE Center. This room is ideal for several reasons:

- It is very small, limiting its use otherwise;

- It has glazed windows that are not transparent and is in a secure, supportive, and private suite of offices;

- It is in a familiar and central location on campus;
- There will be people there to provide orientation, scheduling, monitoring, and cleanup for users;
- Its use will be closely monitored to calculate usage, effectiveness, desirability, etc., for future planning;
- Approved work-life research opportunities exist through usage data, interviews of mothers, etc.

The following provides some preliminary plans for its use. The room will be equipped with a sink, cabinet, a small refrigerator, two to three comfortable chairs, and parenting resources, including a small lending library for new parents. It will be simply but attractively decorated and provide a comfortable, quiet place for a mother to pump milk. Provision of a breast pump is a possibility. Use will be on a first-come, first-served basis, unless scheduling becomes necessary. ADVANCE has a seating area for waiting mothers. When someone is waiting, use will be limited to 20 minutes. We would like to emphasize that providing lactation sites is not a "woman's issue," it is a workplace issue, a health issue, and a parenting issue. We do not see the location of this prototype site in the ADVANCE Center as the answer to the problem, but an excellent first step. For example, evening hours are difficult at this site. We are most eager to provide this service to our URI women, but ADVANCE and the PCOSW hope that once we understand the scope of need, the University will assume the responsibility of providing this important service in other, more general locations on campus (URI ADVANCE, 2006).

The proposal was approved by the President and Campus Planning and Design, and the prototype room was reconfigured (lock on door, sink and cabinet installed by the University, hospital-grade breast pump, and other room furnishings funded by ADVANCE) and opened in 2007. There were several factors that contributed to the success of this first step:

- No institutional commitment was required other than the cost of installing a sink in a small office and replacing a door lock;
- The space was ideally located and was under the jurisdiction of the ADVANCE Center, who was willing to relinquish the space;
- ADVANCE personnel provided room management and oversight, and collected usage data;
- The President was supportive;

A "champion" was involved in the administrative process. The Assistant Director of Campus Planning and Design overseeing space allocation decisions had three young children, and was anticipating a fourth. At least partly because of this personal vantage point, he was sensitive to and supportive of the needs of breastfeeding workers, and was proactive in fast-tracking a minor construction project that might have been considered frivolous by less informed decision-makers and that normally might have taken many more months to complete.

Grant 2: Funding for a Model Lactation Program

Silver and Mederer authored the second grant that was awarded in 2008 by the Elsevier Foundation's New Scholars Program. Like ADVANCE, the New Scholars Program also targets the success of women in STEM, with an emphasis on addressing work-life challenges of junior faculty. The URI award was to develop a lactation policy and program that could be modeled by other universities. We believe the strengths of our proposal included:

- A firm foundation that was laid by the ADVANCE program, which assured success for the next steps and the potential for sustainability;

- The potential to win an institutional Breastfeeding Friendly Workplace award through the Rhode Island Department of Health's Breastfeeding Coalition;

- The plan to embed the program in an array of education and support initiatives (brown bag lunches, literature, workshops, lactation consultant, regional network, etc.);

- A dissemination plan to develop a model program and share it with regional universities and eventually nationally.

> BEST PRACTICE: Through significant grant funding to help retain women in STEM, and additional funding from the Elsevier Foundation's New Scholars Program, URI was able to develop its lactation support program and lactation policy.

During the course of the grant, lactation rooms were established on all three of URI's main campuses, including three on the Kingston campus (this has been increased to five since the grant expired). A lactation policy and guidelines were developed and approved by the administration. A lactation consultant was made available through grant funding, and we engaged in aggressive marketing and publicity to normalize the conversation and increase awareness. These efforts included work-life workshops, events, and newsletters that included information about lactation support, and regular brown bag lunches, some of which were specifically devoted to breastfeeding. It was agreed that all new construction would include a lactation space. URI met the criteria to win a Gold Level Rhode Island Breastfeeding-Friendly Workplace Award, which was presented in a ceremony focused on breastfeeding in the workplace during a campus-wide "Work-Life Day" event that included lactation room tours, an outside speaker, and other offerings. Included in this award was the gift of a second hospital-grade breast pump. A flier for this event can be found in the Appendix. Finally, regional contacts were made and the dissemination program started.

> BEST PRACTICE: URI's lactation policy contains provisions that all new construction of major buildings on campus or significant remodeling of existing buildings include a lactation space.

As part of the dissemination plan, a guidebook was developed by the author that provided lactation program considerations and guidelines specifically geared to colleges and universities. Much of this guidebook, entitled College and University Lactation Programs: Some Additional Considerations, is contained within this chapter. This guidebook is available in PDF format through the URI Work-Life Committee, or can be downloaded from: http://web.uri.edu/worklife/files/LactationPrograms-FINAL.pdf.

Silver partnered with a representative from the Rhode Island Breastfeeding Coalition to begin dissemination of the program model to other Rhode Island colleges and universities. This representative was a registered nurse and lactation consultant, owned a breastfeeding consulting business, and was contracted by the United States Department of Health and Human Services Office on Women's Health to provide the "Business Case for Breastfeeding" (U.S. Department of Health, 2013) to Rhode Island employers. As such, this collaboration proved highly effective, as each partner brought different perspectives and expertise to each meeting. One offered technical and medical expertise, and as an emissary of the Rhode Island Department of Health, offered the potential of small grant funding and of winning an institutional breastfeeding-friendly workplace award available to any organization or business in the state that met award criteria. The other, Silver, focused the conversation on the specific value, mechanics, challenges, and strategies of establishing a lactation program in a college or university setting, and she delivered the guidebook during each of these meetings.

> BEST PRACTICE: Normalizing and validating the topic of breastfeeding in the workplace can be fostered by active marketing, frequent publicity, and regular conversation. Repeated exposure to ideas leads to de-sensitization and more ready acceptance.

We believe the strengths of this second grant program included the following:

- Strong leadership and consistent oversight.

- The creation of a policy and a set of use guidelines (included in Appendix). At URI, when a university policy is proposed, a public comment period is required. We used the opportunity to reach out to all our networks and encourage people to comment in favor of passage of the policy. The comments were overwhelmingly positive, and we have been able to use these comments as evidence for not only the need for a lactation program, but as a way to highlight how important work-life supports are in general for URI employees.

- Extensive marketing and publicity, as indicated above, including brochures and newsletters, and several campus events. Normalizing the topic and de-sensitizing people to it was important to its acceptance as a normal consideration for employees in a workplace.

- Continuing support from the Assistant Director of Campus Planning and Design, who was instrumental in the design of two attractive lactation spaces within new construction in our library and our new College of Pharmacy building.

- Connection and dissemination of the guidebook to Rhode Island colleges and universities.

Most of our ongoing challenges are related to program management and oversight of lactation spaces. First, the institution does not yet support a work-life office or staff member. All work-life efforts are the result of the Work-Life Committee, which originated with the ADVANCE program, and has been co-chaired by Mederer and Silver since 2003. Institutional commitments to maintain an ADVANCE office or person post award did not materialize as the economy and budget challenges worsened at URI, and changes in leadership shifted priorities. Efforts to sustain oversight of the lactation sites and progress beyond these sites remain a volunteer effort by this committee.

Second, space identification remains a continuing challenge, as it is difficult to persuade anyone to offer up space. Securing interest and commitments from those near other lactation sites to help monitor them is a challenge. Placing and maintaining breast pumps is also a challenge as they are valuable and need to be in a secure place. Finally, identifying who "owns" the lactation spaces needed to occur, to ensure they did not revert to storage space or be taken over by other purposes over time. It has recently been agreed that the spaces will all fall under the jurisdiction of the Vice President of Administration (under which the Work-Life Committee operates) rather than under the jurisdiction of each individual building. This requires the committee to maintain oversight.

BEST PRACTICE: Determining who will "own" or maintain oversight over lactation spaces to ensure they remain dedicated spaces is an important consideration, so they do not get usurped by other interested parties over time.

The WLC Approach: A Broad, Societal Perspective and Data-Driven Arguments

The URI Work-Life Committee envisions work-life initiatives as a means to bring about the social changes necessary to meet the diverse needs of our 21st-century workforce. Creating a lactation program was not a difficult or expensive endeavor for URI, in the realm of all the possible initiatives to support women. There are myriad compelling arguments that can be used. The WLC employed the following arguments in support of our program.

From a *moral* perspective, it is contradictory to insist that women offer optimal health opportunities to the next generation of workers and not provide a means to accomplish this. If universities are truly committed to the well being of their employees, they must reach beyond simple solutions to understand and address these cultural contradictions and the underlying barriers that function to sabotage women's progress even while supportive policies, such as paid parental leave, may be in place.

> "I would like to comment on the policy by first saying that I am a mother of three children — all breastfed. In my own experience, the facilities and support available to breastfeeding mothers do have an outcome on length of breastfeeding and job satisfaction. I can speak from experience that having to express breastmilk in a dirty bathroom in a rush is not what new mothers want for their children or from their employer. URI must support this initiative to support working mothers and their families."
>
> -URI employee

From a *legal* perspective, Rhode Island legislation protects a woman's choice to breastfeed by requiring an employer to make "a reasonable effort to provide a private, secure, and sanitary room or other location in close proximity to the work area, other than a toilet stall, where an employee can express her milk or breastfeed her child" (R.I. Gen. Laws § 23-13.2-1). With the passage of the Affordable Care Act's amended Section 7 of the Fair Labor Standards Act, this is now a federal law.

From an *economic* perspective, companies that have adopted breastfeeding support programs have noted cost savings of $3 per $1 invested in breastfeeding support, and experienced less absenteeism, turnover, and lower losses of skilled workers after childbirth, as well as higher employee satisfaction, loyalty, and morale (U.S. Breastfeeding Committee, 2002). Breastfed infants incur significantly lower healthcare costs than do formula-fed infants. Insurers pay at least $3.6 billion each year to treat diseases and conditions preventable by breastfeeding (U.S. Department of Health and Human Services, 2013).

Equity for women provides another compelling argument. Still the predominant caregivers, working-women caregivers experience disproportionate career disadvantages, including slower advancement and threats to job security when caregiving and work responsibilities are pitted against each other. As well, different groups of women are impacted differently by these challenges, making this, in some cases, a class issue as well as a gender issue. Examples include women STEM faculty working in very competitive and traditional male environments; any faculty member whose door is knocked on even when closed with a sign on it; students who have no offices or privacy; lower income staff workers who have no job flexibility to pump milk; and women who, in addition to the many benefits of breastfeeding, are compelled to breastfeed for household economic reasons.

Maintaining a competitive business edge is an argument that resonates broadly. Younger workers, many of whom are women, have higher expectations about what job benefits should be available. Millennial workers are more mobile in their career paths, more dual-centric, prioritizing both life and work responsibilities, and are more insistent on job flexibility and work-life supports when job seeking (Families & Work Institute, 2004). Employers of choice know that to retain a competitive edge, progressive policies must be offered. As the state's flagship university, we aim for the University of Rhode Island to be a leader in this regard. Establishing a lactation program should not be viewed as a benefit or a perk: *it is an effective workplace strategy.*

Changing traditional *norms and workplace cultures* is another vital argument that should be made. Needed is a cultural shift within the workplace that honors employees' life and family responsibilities, and embraces work-life supports while *on* the job, as well as flexibility to be *off* the job to meet family obligations. Without an increased general awareness about the larger benefits to businesses and society of promoting a work-life agenda, and without a shift in individual attitudes and more open, supportive interactions between supervisors and employees, even the best policies cannot be successful. Given our shifting demographics, which includes a marked increase in dual earner couples and eldercare needs, caregiving responsibilities go far beyond what even the best parental leave policies can offer. A workplace culture that supports an employee's caregiving responsibilities throughout the life course is a necessity today.

From a *societal* perspective, there are virtually as many women in the workforce as men, women are increasingly returning to work soon after giving birth, and society strongly encourages new mothers to breastfeed. Today, work and family are no longer separate social institutions—they are interconnected and interdependent. This is clearly a workplace issue more than just a woman's issue: the choices here affect not just mothers and their children, but the next generation of workers, businesses, and society at large.

Finally, the *health* benefits of breastfeeding are well documented, multifold, and encompass significant positive outcomes for mothers and children, as well as the broader scale benefits to healthcare systems and the environment. All major health organizations endorse breastfeeding as the physiological norm for both mothers and infants, as has the Surgeon General (U.S. Department of Health and Human Services, 2011).

> BEST PRACTICE: URI's Work-Life Committee approach is forward thinking in that it exceeds the boundaries of the workplace and considers broad, complex societal issues around breastfeeding.

Creating a Formal Program

Why is it important to design and implement a formal program, as opposed to simply opening a few lactation sites? Trends are clear: 1) mothers today are strongly encouraged to breastfeed for extended periods, 2) most faculty, staff, and student mothers usually return to work or school soon after the birth of their child, and 3) many workplaces are not prepared or willing to accommodate this reality. Too often, the result is that women who do not work in breastfeeding-friendly workplaces stop breastfeeding earlier, or they elect to stay away from work (paid or unpaid) longer, or they endure the stress and inefficiency of finding ways to work or go to school and continue breastfeeding. Numerous anecdotal reports indicate that this stress can be significantly more than is openly acknowledged. Many new breastfeeding mothers returning to work suffer similar pressures to the ones suffered by this graduate student:

> "Breastfeeding certainly wasn't anything I could talk about. When I returned to graduate school within days of giving birth to my daughter, I would have to walk to my car, leave the campus, drive down a back road with my Playmate cooler and breast pump, find a quiet stopping place, pump in my car, all the time nervously scanning the road for passersby, return to campus, try to find another parking place, and go back to work, feeling somehow embarrassed and like I'd just committed some kind of misdemeanor" (Personal communication, URI graduate student, 2008).

Fundamentally, a formal program helps to validate the importance of lactation support as a workplace issue, ensures that all employees and supervisors become educated about and adhere to a consistent set of rules, and promotes equitable access to services for all employees. A formal lactation program can challenge traditional mainstream tendencies to render invisible the differential impact caretaking challenges can have on women's career advancement. It legitimizes a practice that is expected to occur somehow invisibly by women, and normalizes a sensitive topic within a campus community, recognizing it as a workplace/workforce—rather than a personal—issue. It formally acknowledges the intersection of work and family in today's workplace and can, therefore, promote cultural change in a department and an institution, especially as it benefits all breastfeeding mothers, including faculty, staff, and students.

It is important to realize that the need for lactation resources may not be openly evident. Many Human Resources departments do not attend to this topic because they do not see the need. This became clear to us as we visited other Rhode Island schools. *It should not be assumed, just because there have been few requests for lactation time or there is little awareness of the number of women who would benefit, that the need is not there.* As well, providing a lactation program carries a highly positive symbolic value and speaks loudly about an employer's desire to support the work-life needs of its employees. The many comments about the new lactation policy from URI employees, most of whom would likely never even need to use lactation resources, attest to this. *It is a low-cost, high-return initiative employers can offer.*

URI created a formal program that was composed of four general components: 1) a policy, 2) a set of usage guidelines, 3) identification of facilities, and 4) education and awareness initiatives. The following four sections include some "how to" program guidelines outlined in the aforementioned guidebook: *College and University Lactation Programs: Some Additional Considerations.*

BEST PRACTICE: URI was wise to include provisions to formalize their lactation program. By implementing a policy, a set of usage guidelines, a provision for lactation space in new and renovated facilities, and education and awareness initiatives, they provided their program with permanency regardless of changes in oversight.

Part One: Create a Policy

Why? There are several reasons why a formal policy is important. They include the following:

- **Visible Institutional Support**. We know that many women stop breastfeeding early to avoid the challenges of returning to work and trying to express milk away from home. The myriad positive impacts of continuing to breastfeed to mother, infant, and society are well documented. Establishing a formal policy is a strong institutional statement of support.

- **Encourage Fairness and Transparency**. Formal policy creation is important to ensure fair and consistent application of practices across supervisors/chairs and categories of employees. Ad hoc or case-by-case management of lactation requests will be inconsistent and non-transparent, be wasteful of time and energy, and will invite inequities and employee resentment.

- **Inclusivity Across Job Categories**. Many categories of staff employees may not have the level of flexibility that faculty often enjoy. And even faculty (and students) may not feel they have the time or appropriate space to express milk. Establishing a policy is an equity issue.

- **Encourage Consistent Supervisory Support**. Supervisors/ chairs will vary in their level of understanding and support for women who need time to express breastmilk. Without a formal, visible policy in place, many employees may not know to ask for time to express milk, or will worry about negative job repercussions if they do ask. While a policy alone may not be enough to encourage use, it is an important first step. Just because there may not have been many requests for lactation resources doesn't mean they haven't been needed—employees may be just "making do" on their own or stopping breastfeeding altogether.

- **Normalize the Topic**. Lactation support can be a sensitive subject for some, and it is important that the topic be broached openly and regularly to normalize it, rather than to marginalize it as a "woman's issue," shrouded in secrecy and even embarrassment. Some women and some supervisors, particularly male supervisors, may be uncomfortable discussing this topic, and making it a normal, expected issue to review prior to or when a new mother returns to work is important.

- **Correcting a Cultural Contradiction**. There is a cultural contradiction surrounding breastfeeding in the workplace. That is, while new mothers experience strong societal encouragement for breastfeeding and are increasingly returning to work for economic and professional reasons, they are often faced with a lack of formal support for breastfeeding in the workplace.

> "I think this is a great policy. It surely will help breastfeeding mothers on campus. This policy will encourage breastfeeding. A mother does not need to make a choice between giving up breastfeeding and giving up full time status. Thank you!"
>
> -URI employee

How? The policy creation process varies by institution, falling along a continuum between straightforward to very cumbersome or not feasible. The following guiding principles may be useful:

- **Understand the formal procedural steps** your institution uses to establish policy. Introduce the idea to the administrators who would be involved in the decision-making process at your institution to encourage buy-in.

- **Identify influential individuals** and/or groups on campus who are supportive of this initiative to co-author or otherwise support the policy request.

- **Carefully select the author(s)** of any introductory letters, as well as the policy request, especially if resistance is expected. Human Resources may or may not be the most effective source, depending on the institution. Women's commissions, equity councils, diversity officers, etc., may be more successful. A work-life director or office is obviously another source.

- **Develop a rationale**, or case statement, referring to some or all of the arguments described above, such as state law and the business case for breastfeeding. Also include examples of peer institutions' programs and an estimate of the projected need at your institution.

- **Utilize the larger agenda of work-life balance**, workplace flexibility, equity, and diversity, to frame your request. The rationale for promoting workplace flexibility is readily available from many sources. The URI Work-Life website has language about the current work-life movement, as well as links to other websites and resources: http://www.uri.edu/worklife.

- **Rather than a women's issue**, frame lactation support as a workplace and workforce issue. Today, there are as many women in the workforce as men, and dual earner households are the norm. Supporting breastfeeding is supporting the next generation of workers; it is *not* simply an accommodation for women.

- **Develop a policy statement** and an accompanying set of guidelines.

- If the policy approval process includes a **public comment period**, take advantage of this by encouraging your networks to respond. Comments will likely be overwhelmingly positive. Track comments and use them to your advantage.

- **Have a management plan**, including a timeline and a person responsible for promoting the program, collecting data, overseeing facilities, and ensuring sustainability.

- **Have a marketing plan,** including literature, websites, brown bag lunches, announcements, visits to department meetings, etc. Consider making it part of a work-life website (see www.uri. edu/worklife, as an example).

> "I think that this and the parental leave policy that went into effect a few years ago are exactly what this community needs to get us heading into the right direction. The right direction being our development into a family-friendly community, one which is aware of and supports the challenges we all face outside the workplace."
>
> -URI employee

Part Two: Develop Guidelines

Guidelines generally should include information about how lactation break time is managed for employees and students, the importance of supervisory support for flexible scheduling, how an employee's needs must be respected, but also fairly balanced with the needs of the organization, and where additional resources and advocacy can be attained. These points are briefly outlined below.

Supervisors and employees should work together to arrange mutually agreeable break times, typically two to three times a day, paid or unpaid. Employers should become familiar with the amended Section 7 of the Fair Labor Standards Act regarding appropriate break time, as well as any corresponding state law, if one exists, as its provisions will take precedence if it provides more protection for nursing mothers (U.S. Department of Labor, 2010). While this may be unnecessary for faculty or students who have more flexibility, adopting a request form for staff employees that includes guidance on how to negotiate a conversation with a supervisor can be very helpful.

While break time can be paid or unpaid, it is advised that flexible scheduling be considered where possible to make up time, rather than penalizing nursing mothers by withholding pay. Descriptions of flexible work options are available at many work-life websites, and can also be found at the URI Work-Life website (www.uri.edu/worklife).

Supervisors/chairs are expected and encouraged to respond positively and supportively to an employee's request for lactation break time, and no negative job repercussions should result. However, it is also assumed, and should be emphasized, that no serious disruption of the institution's operations will occur. An effective negotiation of lactation break time should result in a win-win for everyone.

It should not usually be necessary to provide break times for students. Generally, students may have more flexibility with their break times and should be able to use these times for expressing milk or nursing. In some cases, however, tight schedules may certainly justify schedule negotiations on an individual basis between professor and student. Students who need additional flexibility are encouraged to speak with their professors about this, and also to access whatever work-life resources or advocacy is available at their institution.

It is important to provide an avenue for employees and students to get more information, or to voice concerns, especially if they are not getting supervisory support for their requests. An advocate, a mentor, perhaps someone in Human Resources, or a work-life specialist should be available. *This issue is often and too easily avoided by women who encounter resistance.* This may be particularly true in male-dominated domains, such as in the sciences and engineering (Xu & Martin, 2011), and in units managed by supervisors who are openly or passively resistant.

Part Three: Identify Facilities

Unlike many businesses, campuses are usually large and spread out. Identifying several locations that do not require long walks for women who have limited break time or time between classes is important. While it is understandable that some programs may grow slowly over time as sites are identified and space is negotiated, an ideal rule-of-thumb is to provide enough sites so that no more than a five-minute walk is required.

Many institutions, such as URI, start small with a pilot space and expand as other spaces are identified. Space is usually at a premium at a university, and negotiating lactation space can be especially challenging. Securing space may require finding an advocate in each building who has some influence over its use. The location may be the place the employee normally works if there is adequate privacy, cleanliness, and is comfortable for the employee. Areas such as restrooms are not considered appropriate spaces for lactation purposes, unless the restroom is equipped with a separate, designated lactation room, such as might be available in a large locker room.

It should be a program priority to campaign to have all new construction or renovation projects include a small lactation space. Facilities can be very simple if resources or management personnel are limited, and can include only a small, clean, private space with a chair, small table, a lockable door, and an electrical outlet for a breast pump. Access to nearby running water is important. When resources and oversight permits, spaces can include a hospital-grade breast pump and a sink. Some facilities offer a refrigerator for milk storage, although there are differing positions on this, as there may be risks involved in leaving milk in a public refrigerator, such as tampering and contamination of stored milk. Where breast pumps are provided, spaces must be managed, cleaned, and secured. Other considerations include locating spaces that are open long hours, such as a student union building or a library, for those remaining late on campus, and offering a small "new parent" resource library in a location that has oversight.

Program managers should think long term about how responsible oversight will occur. While labeling the space as a "Lactation Room" is preferred as a means to normalize and validate this activity, it could also be identified as a Mother's Room or a Privacy Room or similar, with a lactation logo to further identify its purpose. Choosing an alternative label could expand its use to any employee or student who needs private time for medical or health reasons, which might promote more general "buy-in" if there is significant resistance. However, this alternative should be weighed against the negative impact of continuing to disguise lactation support and the potential for inappropriate use of the space.

Where feasible, program facilitators could consider data collection to provide support for expanding facilities in the future. Short surveys and sign-in sheets can provide some indication of usage, though this is difficult to track in unmonitored spaces. How and whether to schedule room usage is also a consideration, depending on level of use, oversight options, and data collection considerations.

Conclusion: Promoting Broad Support

The most challenging aspect of starting a lactation program may be enlisting the broad support of supervisors, chairs, and administrators. It is naïve to assume that all supervisors understand, support, or are comfortable addressing this particular issue, or work-life balance issues in general. Likewise, women are often reluctant to come forward with a request for lactation time for a variety of reasons, including lack of understanding about their rights, embarrassment, or fear of negative job repercussions.

The issue should be framed within the larger context of work-life balance, workplace flexibility, workplace equity, and the changing nature of our workforce. *A lactation program is not an accommodation for women; it is a contemporary workforce issue and a community health issue.* Normalizing the conversation by making it a frequently addressed issue will help. Brown bag lunches, literature dissemination, website links, talks, press releases, work-life workshops, new parent support groups, etc., are all methods for educating the community and should appear regularly. Identifying a liaison or spokesperson in each college/unit/division is a good means to broaden support, information dissemination, and general awareness.

Chairs and supervisors need to understand the subtle barriers to advancement that exist for working mothers in highly competitive academic environments. First, for faculty, providing lactation support is a promotion and tenure equity issue, because women's prime childbearing years typically overlap with the tenure track years. The challenges of juggling the demands of a new baby, continuing to breastfeed while returning to work, and remaining competitive on the tenure track disadvantage women over men. Next, for many staff workers, providing lactation support is an equity issue and a socioeconomic issue, as hourly workers typically have greater constraints on their time. They should not be denied the same opportunities to advance their careers, their health, and their family's health that other employees may have. Finally, student populations are increasingly diverse, including older students returning to college or graduate school. Providing facilities for new student mothers is important as well.

Fundamentally, the active promotion of a "culture of coverage" in departments and units should be paramount (Mederer & Silver, 2011). In addition to supervisors, co-workers also need to be educated about these issues. Supervisors and chairs should model and encourage co-worker support and work coverage when needed, not just for lactation breaks, but for a wide variety of reasons a co-worker would need to be away from work due to family, personal, or health concerns. As our workplace and workforce evolve, the emphasis should be squarely directed at the reality that every worker will have caregiving challenges at some point in time, whether for themselves, their children, and/or their aging parents. A culture of coverage embraces the adage, "what goes around, comes around." Lactation support must be included in that repertoire.

References

Families and Work Institute (2004). Gender and generation in the workplace: An issue brief. Waltham, MA: American Business Collaboration.

Ginther, D. (2006). The economics of gender differences in employment outcomes in academia. In Committee on Maximizing the potential of Women in Academic Science and Engineering, et al. *Biological, Social and Organizational Components of Success for Women in Academic Science and Engineering.* Washington DC: National Academies Press.

Mederer, H. & Silver, B. (2011). *Workplace flexibility and faculty success: What a chair needs to know.* URI Chairs' Workshop presentation, University of Rhode Island, Kingston, RI. Retrieved from http://www.uri.edu/worklife/_assets/ Resources/Presentations/Chairs%27%20Work-Life%20workshop%20HM.pdf

U.S. Breastfeeding Committee. (2002). *Workplace breastfeeding support* [Issue Paper]. Raleigh, NC: U. S. Breastfeeding Committee.

U.S. Department of Health and Human Services, Office on Women's Health. (2013). *The business case for breastfeeding.* Retrieved from http://www. womenshealth.gov/breastfeeding/government-in-action/business-case-for- breastfeeding/

U.S. Department of Health and Human Services. (2011). *The surgeon general's call to action to support breastfeeding.* Retrieved from http://www. surgeongeneral.gov/library/calls/breastfeeding/index.html

U.S. Department of Labor. (2010). *Fact Sheet #73: Break time for nursing mothers under the FLSA.* Retrieved from: http://www.dol.gov/whd/regs/ compliance/whdfs73.htm

University of Rhode Island (URI) ADVANCE Program. (2006). *Proposal for a URI lactation center.* Retrieved from: http://www.uri.edu/advance/files/pdf/ Lactation%20Program%20Rationale%20final.pdf

Xu, Y. J., & Martin, C. L. (2011). Gender differences in STEM disciplines: From the aspects of informal professional networking and faculty career development. *Gender Issues, 28,* 134-154.

Chapter Four
Long Ago But Not Far Away: A Pioneering Effort for Campus-Wide Lactation Accommodation at University of California Davis

Barbara Ashby

The Breastfeeding Support Program at the University of California Davis began in 1995, long before family-friendly agendas, advocacy, and the law pushed lactation accommodation to the forefront of workplace practices. Core to UC Davis' robust portfolio of WorkLife resources and services, it is open to all campus affiliates (nursing faculty, staff, students, and their spouses/domestic partners) and visitors. Four components provide a solid infrastructure—policy, facilities, education, and support—with an overarching goal to facilitate women's return to work/school after maternity leave and to foster an encouraging and supportive environment toward successful continuation of breastfeeding. Administered centrally by the WorkLife office, the UC Davis Breastfeeding Support Program provides hospital-grade breast pumps in nearly fifty dedicated lactation sites, no-cost services of a board certified lactation consultant, quarterly classes, monthly support group meetings, and a research and referral newsletter. UC Davis' success in building a best practice program comes from its comprehensive and integrated approach to lactation accommodation.

Advancing the University Vision and Mission

The University of California Davis is located in northern California between San Francisco and Sacramento, the state capitol. A member of the Association of American Universities, UC Davis is comprised of four colleges, six professional schools, a medical center and health system enrolling 33,000-plus students (54% of whom are female) and employing roughly 17,000 academic, professional, and support staff (59% of whom are female). It is the largest of the ten campuses in the public University of California system, encompassing 5,300 acres and more than 1,000 buildings. UC Davis was founded in 1905 as a land-grant university, an institution of higher education built upon public lands donated by Congress to states under the Morrill Acts of 1862 and 1890. The purpose of land-grant universities was to teach agriculture, science, engineering, and military science, in addition to classical studies, so that working-class students could obtain a liberal and practical education.

The scope and goals of the Breastfeeding Support Program align with and advance the University's mission of teaching, research, and public service driven by its land-grant heritage. The campus *Vision of Excellence* states: "The mission of UC Davis, as a comprehensive research university, is the generation, advancement, dissemination, and application of knowledge to advancing the human condition throughout our communities and around the world. In this, UC Davis is committed to developing and sustaining leading programs." One area of renown is the study of human milk, lactation, and infant nutrition. The UC Davis Breastfeeding Support Program exemplifies the translation and application of such research to best practices that support social responsibility and a sustainable global environment. The *Vision of Excellence* identifies six primary goals and associated metrics:

- Foster a vibrant community of learning and scholarship;
- Drive innovation at the frontiers of knowledge;
- Embrace global issues;
- Nurture a sustainable future and propel economic vitality;
- Champion health, education, access, and opportunity;
- Cultivate a culture of organizational excellence, effectiveness, and stewardship.

The Breastfeeding Support Program promotes health, wellness, and enhanced quality of life for children and families. It enables women to return to school/work at the University while continuing to breastfeed exclusively and longer in keeping with the objectives of Healthy People 2020 and recommendations of the American Academy of Pediatrics. The program is among "the number, quality, and availability of educational and healthy living resources, community partnerships, and referral mechanisms for healthcare, nutrition, and community wellbeing" that represent achievement of the University's vision.

In addition, the *Vision of Excellence* affirms UC Davis' "abiding commitment to diversity, as represented in our community and in our

perspectives, as foundational elements of our excellence. We shall…
be resolute in advancing inclusion and equity in our community." The
Breastfeeding Support Program increases the community's understanding
of the importance of breastfeeding from many perspectives and
promotes a culture of respect and encouragement for work-life
effectiveness.

> BEST PRACTICE: Considering breastfeeding as a foundational element of the
> Vision of Excellence, the UC Davis Breastfeeding Support Program took root,
> strengthened, and grew steadily in alignment with the institution's mission and
> guiding principles.

Engaging a Diverse Group to Create a Model Program

The inception of the Breastfeeding Support Program began in
1994 with the Chancellor's Administrative Advisory Committee on
Child Care, comprised of faculty, staff, and students charged with
advising the Associate Vice Chancellor of Human Resources on
programs and policies to meet the childcare needs of the campus
community; assessing and articulating concerns, services, and funding;
and providing a campus forum for issues. During one of its monthly
meetings, a graduate student from the department of Nutrition addressed
the committee about the need for breastfeeding support on campus. She
was working in a major laboratory for lactation research and noticed
that many of the women in their clinical studies were asking if they could
borrow the breast pumps used in that work. Women also stopped in at
the department office to inquire if there was an accommodating place
to use their own breast pumps. The health benefits of breastmilk were
well documented, but there was no system in place to accommodate
lactating mothers. Campus women who wanted to continue to provide
their babies with breastmilk after returning to work/school often would
resort to pumping in their cars or a bathroom stall, or abandoning the
effort altogether.

The committee recommended action and the Associate Vice
Chancellor of Human Resources tasked the campus Childcare
Coordinator, who was staff to the committee, with finding ways to
provide lactation support at UC Davis. The Childcare Coordinator
position reported jointly to the Associate Vice Chancellor of Human
Resources and the Director of Community and Student Housing,
facilitating straightforward collaboration between administrative and
student services. It was the kernel from which future family services
evolved and eventually grew into the comprehensive WorkLife office
that manages the Breastfeeding Support Program today. Further synergy
and commitment came from personal and professional experience.

Several years prior, the Coordinator had been a graduate student and new mother at UC Davis who had to express milk for her first-born in conditions that were far from ideal. Over the course of one year, the Coordinator researched and developed models for service delivery, explored real estate for lactation sites, established partnerships with numerous departments, implemented a communications strategy, and launched the UC Davis Breastfeeding Support Program.

Nearly two decades later, the program has become a valued attribute of campus life and recognized resource to the local community. In addition to the Chancellor's Administrative Advisory Committee on Child Care, it has the respect and advocacy of the Faculty WorkLife Advisors chaired by the Vice Provost for Academic Affairs and the Status of Women at Davis Administrative Advisory Committee sponsored by the Associate Executive Vice Chancellor of Campus Community Relations. In 2009, the UC System-wide Advisory Committee on the Status of Women, Work/Life Subcommittee, recommended the Davis Breastfeeding Support Program as the model for the other nine UC campuses. The UC Davis Breastfeeding Support Program has earned numerous awards for work-life effectiveness and health promotion:

- Innovative Excellence Award from the Alliance of Work-Life Professionals, 2002;

- Mother-Baby Friendly Workplace Statewide Award from the California Task Force on Youth and Workplace Wellness, 2005;

- Mother-Baby Friendly Workplace Countywide Award from the Community Breastfeeding Coalition of Yolo County, 2005-2008;

- Best Practice Model for Higher Education from the U.S. Department of Health and Human Services Office on Women's Health, 2012.

> BEST PRACTICE: Gaining the interest and support of campus committees and interest groups responsible for work-life, diversity, and inclusion matters promoted awareness and recognition of the UC Davis Breastfeeding Support Program as a community asset.

Creating a Cutting Edge Initiative for the Community

As a cutting edge initiative with roots in the multi-constituent Chancellor's Administrative Advisory Committee on Child Care, both the development and ongoing expansion efforts of the UC Davis Breastfeeding Support Program have made it a point to serve the entire campus community (nursing faculty, staff, students, and their spouses/domestic partners) and not solely employees. In keeping with the University's mission of public service, even conference attendees and visiting colleagues are welcome to use the lactation sites, while local residents may attend the educational classes and support group meetings space permitting.

Because many members of an academic community often live away from family, having an institutional support system is important to personal wellbeing and professional success. In *Better Educating Our New Breadwinners: Creating opportunities for all women to succeed in the workforce (Mason, 2009),* Mary Ann Mason, professor and former dean of the graduate division at the University of California Berkeley, indicates that more women with family responsibilities are attending all levels of post-secondary education, but they need family-friendly policies and practices to complete their degrees. Student families face stress as they balance academics, employment, child rearing, and rising costs of living and education. Breastfeeding is estimated to save about $1,500 in formula costs for one year. Access to private space, efficient breast pumps for milk expression, and support to meet their breastfeeding goals is especially helpful for students whose time and resources are stretched.

Case in point: When Julie was pregnant with her son, she was also confronting some very difficult events that affected her personally and professionally. At that time she was a third year doctoral student in the Agriculture and Environmental Chemistry Graduate Group at UC Davis and considered taking an extended leave from her program. Although she was faced with challenging circumstances, Julie made the decision to return to school because she felt that UC Davis' supportive resources (including her professor, colleagues, and classmates) *wanted* her to continue. Julie then found out about the Breastfeeding Support Program through the Women's Resource and Research Center on campus and realized how much support the campus provides for new mothers. Since her partner lives away from home during the week, Julie found the support and encouragement she needed to continue her life as a new breastfeeding mom who also worked and pursued her Ph.D. Julie says that she doesn't know "if I would have been able to come back to school if it wasn't for that program."

The decision to extend the Breastfeeding Support Program to spouses and domestic partners of employees and students was one of equity and inclusion. It eliminated what could have been considered a discriminatory benefit, garnered the support of the male population and LGBTQ community, and advanced the University's commitment to being a model employer promoting family-friendly policies and practices for work-life effectiveness, particularly regarding wellness and dependent care.

Case in point: "My wife (who does not work at UC Davis) and I *[male, assistant professor]* recently had our first child—this is an exciting new adventure for us, and also a bit overwhelming. My wife has participated in the Breastfeeding Support Group, and together we met with the campus lactation consultant for help resolving some breastfeeding challenges. Both the support group and the consultation helped us quite a lot. We are very grateful that this support was available for us. UC Davis and the city of Davis are great places to work and live...The Breastfeeding Support Program at UC Davis contributes directly to this."

BEST PRACTICE: UC Davis made an important move by positioning the program as more than a workplace accommodation, but as a breastfeeding support for students and spouses/domestic partners, as well as employees.

Partnerships: Partnering Makes a Difference

Launching the UC Davis Breastfeeding Support Program was a pioneering effort to find and convert spaces and to build the infrastructure with minimal resources. Goodwill was ample; funding was not. The solution was to take an organic approach and form partnerships with various administrative departments that could provide what was needed. Custodial Services identified anterooms in women's lounges. Facilities Services donated labor and materials to renovate them. Student Housing supplied furniture. Leveraging the UC Davis Medical Center's durable medical equipment contract with a major breast pump manufacturer enabled the lactation sites to be equipped with hospital-grade, multi-user pumps. Anything more than a manual breast pump was expensive and the rental pumps were bulky and cumbersome to transport. The Bookstore agreed to sell the personal attachment kits at a price just above their cost. The Student Health Center hosted twice-monthly registration and orientation sessions. University Communications frequently featured the program in its publications, including a spotlight on public television.

BEST PRACTICE: A key partnership with the University bookstore made it possible for UC Davis program participants to purchase the personal attachment kits for pumps at a discounted price at convenient locations on campus.

Partnership with the UC Davis Foods for Health Institute reinforces the Breastfeeding Support Program's practical application of the University's mission and *Vision of Excellence* regarding teaching, research, and public service. Advancements in the Foods for Health Institute's Milk Bioactives and Functional Glycobiology studies enable the Breastfeeding Support Program to disseminate the most current research findings about the benefits of human milk and breastfeeding, thereby promoting awareness and public good. Faculty members serve as consultants and contribute to the program's quarterly newsletter. The Institute also provides student interns who assist with administrative tasks, as well as the set-up and maintenance of lactation sites. Their inspections of the lactation sites are important for maintaining the cleanliness and integrity of the rooms and addressing issues that arise.

> BEST PRACTICE: A partnership with academic researchers from the UC Davis Foods for Health Institute facilitates the dissemination of the most current research findings.

The Women's Resources and Research Center contributes meeting space for educational classes and support groups. The on-campus child development centers inform parents about the program and welcome mothers to breastfeed their enrolled infants and toddlers directly at the centers whenever possible. One of the centers has provided children's artwork to hang in some lactation sites. Grants from the county First 5 Yolo Children and Families Commission and the Venture Club have funded purchases of breast pumps in keeping with their organizational missions to support women, children, and families. Although many nursing mothers now own portable pumps, provision of hospital-grade equipment is still a very popular aspect of the UC Davis Breastfeeding Support Program, as it makes milk expression more effective and efficient, and saves participants the effort of toting their own.

> BEST PRACTICE: UC Davis capitalized on partnerships with administrative and academic departments, local social service agencies, and philanthropic groups, which helped them to build and strengthen their lactation program's infrastructure.

Building the Inventory of Sites to Accommodate Demand

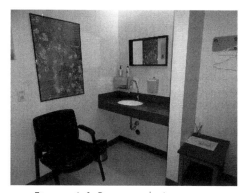

Figure 4.1 Room with Access to Running Water

Within a year of the initial idea being raised, three dedicated lactation sites had been established on the central UC Davis campus. Over time more spaces followed based on documented usage and demand. Signage in each site reminded women to register for the program and to login and out each time they used a site, as funding and expansion depended upon proving the need. That practice of documenting usage also had the added benefit of making it easier for participants to self-monitor their usage and plan their milk expression breaks accordingly. Occasionally, arrangements were made through Disability Management Services for other building occupants to use a room for medical accommodations. For example, a staff member recovering from a back injury would take her rest breaks in the quiet privacy of the lactation site conveniently located in her department. Nursing mothers retained priority, however. This compromise established goodwill and minimized battles over real estate.

In 2001, California Assembly Bill 1025 was passed requiring employers to provide access to a private space "within close proximity" to an employee's work area. That caveat facilitated collaboration with campus Architects and Engineers to expand the availability and accessibility of lactation sites across campus. In 2004, a five-minute walking rule was established (calculated at two miles per hour or about 800 feet), a study was done to map and identify additional site locations, and renovations ensued to convert storage rooms, custodial supply closets, offices, and portions of locker rooms to clean, safe, comfortable, and dedicated lactation sites. Every attempt was made to locate each site near a sink with hot, running water (Figure 4.1). This project resulted in a campus standard for design and construction requiring a lactation room "in every major new campus building" unless waived by the WorkLife office.

> BEST PRACTICE: To assure availability and access to lactation sites across campus, a five-minute walking rule (calculated at two miles per hour or about 800 feet) was implemented at UC Davis.

Lactation accommodation is a recognized element of space planning at UC Davis. There are almost 50 readily-available, easily-accessible lactation sites within close proximity of work/study areas and classrooms, even in the most remote corners of campus and in commercial property the university leases from the local community. Program participants are free to choose and use whatever sites work best for them. Students, whose time on campus is nomadic by nature, often frequent multiple sites, while office-based employees tend to use the rooms within or closest to their worksite.

The campus design standard states that at a minimum all lactation rooms shall have:

- A lavatory for hand and equipment washing.
- Open counter space at lavatory.

84

- Space for a chair or bench and small table to place pump on. Chair should have washable surface, arms, good back support.

- A U-bolt shall be installed in either the floor or wall near the pump table to attach a cable for securing the pump equipment.

- A duplex electrical receptacle (preferably near chair and table).

- Privacy (i.e., no windows to the public).

- Adequate signage for easy location within a building.

- Occupied/Unoccupied Signage on exterior of the door.

- A lock for privacy—no keys, keypad preferred.

- A tack board or other wall-mounted system to provide informational flyers and sign-in sheet.

- Natural day lighting.

- A coat hook.

Designers use this checklist to comply with the campus standard. Construction Project Managers review the lactation room layouts with the WorkLife office to be sure they meet program needs. All sites are stocked with disinfectant wipes for quick cleanup to maintain a healthy environment. Some sites include lockers (Figure 4.2). The sites provide a haven away from interruptions and are more conducive to the milk letdown reflex (Figures 4.3 – 4.6).

Case in point: One faculty member who participated in the program remarked that the rooms "are fantastic in terms of being able to maintain pumping. Even though I have a private office, I share the space, so the lactation room allows me to go into a quiet place and just think about my baby."

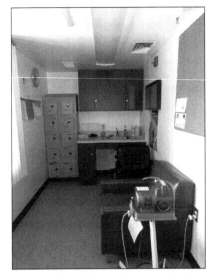
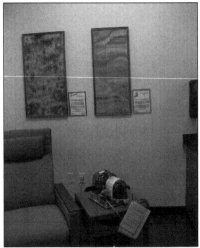
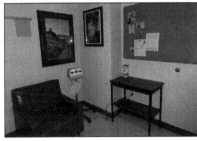
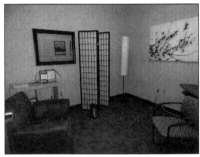
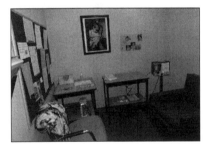

Figures 4.5 – 4.6 Lactation Rooms
(left to right)

Providing a Comprehensive Program Involves Education and Support

Since its inception the UC Davis Breastfeeding Support Program has offered free-of-charge the professional services of an international board certified lactation consultant (IBCLC) in recognition of the fact that a woman's ability to meet her breastfeeding goals often depends on the support she receives. The first consultant was on staff at the

UC Davis Medical Center where she provided inpatient services as a registered nurse in the Labor and Delivery unit. Although only funded for ten hours a month with the Breastfeeding Support Program, her expertise and contributions left a lasting impact and legacy. The lactation consultant lead bimonthly registration and orientation sessions that included an array of materials instructing moms on how to use and get the best results from the breast pumps located in the lactation sites; safely handle, store, and re-feed expressed milk; create a pumping schedule; maintain milk production; and address breast health issues that may arise. Her focus was to assist women with the transition back to work/school from maternity leave and refer them to local La Leche League groups, community educators, and/or medical practitioners for more individualized assistance and care. She encouraged program participants to build relationships with each other by displaying their babies' photos in the sites, exchanging thoughts through a communal journal available in each site, and attending periodic potluck lunches that the program hosted. Most sites contained two chairs and several were equipped with two breast pumps, leading some women to take their milk expression breaks together and provide support for each other. Eventually, a formal support group facilitated by the lactation consultant was formed. The group provided information, advice, camaraderie, encouragement, and practical wisdom through all stages of breastfeeding.

Steady increases in program enrollment and high marks on annual client evaluations made the case for additional resources. A lending library of books and videos was established. Expectant parents were encouraged to join the program during pregnancy to learn about the postpartum experience and role of breastfeeding in early child development. Lactation consultation was in demand, especially in challenging situations, such as twins, premature or sick infants, or infants with special needs. Other mothers needed clinical support to address poor latch, inadequate milk transfer or supply, or nipple or breast pain. Early success at initial breastfeeding increased the likelihood of women continuing to breastfeed after returning to work/school and striving to attain the American Academy of Pediatrics recommendation of six months exclusive breastfeeding. Access to an attentive, knowledgeable professional with helpful, practical advice eased the adjustment period, especially when there were difficulties.

Case in point: One doctoral student who took advantage of this benefit lauded the lactation consultant as "not only more accessible than some of my doctors, but her knowledge has often been a lot more detailed."

There is a lactation consultant on staff ten hours per week to teach education classes (preparing for breastfeeding, balancing breastfeeding with work/school, and weaning), lead support groups, recommend content for the program's website, and consult in person, by phone, or by email with families who have simple questions through serious concerns. In addition, the lactation consultant oversees publication of a quarterly newsletter by the program as another resource to help women minimize and overcome barriers to successful breastfeeding. The newsletter answers frequently asked questions, offers strategies for preventing and managing common breastfeeding problems, and highlights current research findings and evidence-based practices.

Secondly, there is a strong sense of connection and community among the program participants. A lot of empathy, comfort, sharing, and learning is exchanged between expectant, new, and more experienced parents dealing with similar and often challenging circumstances. Attending support group meetings normalizes the process of breastfeeding and eases some of the stress new mothers feel as they hear from other women whose babies have gone through and moved beyond developmental phases. Participation during pregnancy and maternity leave creates a solid foundation that provides the most benefits to both the families and the University. The best testimony to the program's return on investment is participants returning with their second and third children. Frequent comments from program participants show appreciation for the guidance and encouragement they give each other and reflect a sense of completion and giving back to a cause outside of their professional focus. Upon leaving the program, these families take with them a dedication to promoting supportive environments for breastfeeding.

> BEST PRACTICE: The UC Davis Breastfeeding Support Program demonstrates the importance of providing lactation support, not just milk expression spaces.

It is important to keep in mind that positive job satisfaction correlates with achieving breastfeeding goals. The Patient Protection and Affordable Care Act requires healthcare plans to provide breastfeeding supplies and consultation. Workplace lactation programs can do more, like provide information and refer women to free resources. There is little need for workplace accommodation if women give up on breastfeeding before returning from maternity leave. This focus is so important to the mothers they serve that they return after their next babies are born.

Create Awareness and Increase Utilization

Getting the word out about the UC Davis Breastfeeding Support Program before the proliferation of electronic media took a grassroots effort as well. It relied extensively on existing vehicles, such as new employee and student orientations, maternity benefits counseling, the childcare information and referral network, tabling at resource fairs, memo lines on payroll statements, articles in the campus and local newspapers, and a directive to deans, department chairs, and administrative officers. And, of course, lots of fliers were posted across campus. The on-site child development centers included information about the program in their information packets for new and expectant parents. The program's lactation consultant presented at the quarterly workshops on pregnancy in the workplace taught by Human Resources. Word-of-mouth from other program participants and local La Leche League leaders provided powerful endorsements.

In addition to the early communications methods, most of which are still in use, mass marketing is facilitated through the WorkLife website. A standing column in an electronic newsletter published monthly by the WorkLife office features breastfeeding classes and support group events. The footprint has been expanded through collaboration with the county Women, Infants, and Children (WIC) agency and the Breastfeeding Coalition, which sponsors the Community Breastfeeding Warmline. Local hospital labor and delivery nurses refer patients. Most importantly, policy requires supervisors to inform pregnant employees.

Law and Policy Help Mothers Meet Their Breastfeeding Goals

A campus directive to deans, department chairs, and administrative officers announced the launch of the UC Davis Breastfeeding Support Program in 1995 and established an expectation of encouragement for participation. After the passage of California law requiring workplace accommodation, a second directive in 2002 clarified the University's obligation and commitment to accommodate employees and students who were nursing mothers.

In 2008, a formal lactation accommodation policy was fully vetted and adopted into UC Davis' personnel policies and procedures manual to ensure fair and consistent practices. It states that the "University of California is committed to providing a supportive environment that enables employees and students to express their milk in private, in an appropriate space, and in reasonable proximity to their work and study areas." Details address break times, flexible work arrangements, facilities, identification, and support, including supervisor's responsibilities. "Upon notification by an employee of her pregnancy and intent to breastfeed, the supervisor will discuss lactation options in preparation for her return to work after the birth of her baby.

The supervisor will advise the employee of her right to a reasonable amount of break time and a private location to express breastmilk. The supervisor will inform the employee of the resources available through the campus Breastfeeding Support Program."

Workplace flexibility arrangements are also covered under personnel policies. Human Resources provide guidelines, checklists, and agreement forms to assist with development and implementation.

The University of California issued a lactation accommodation policy for its ten-campus system. In his introductory letter of July 2013 to the Chancellors, President Mark Yudof stated: "As part of our commitment to a workplace culture supportive of family caregiving responsibilities and in recognition of the importance and benefits of breastfeeding for both mothers and their infants, the University established the staff policy on Accommodations for Nursing Mothers." A copy of the policy and letter are included in the Appendix.

Results of a recent survey of UC Davis Breastfeeding Support Program participants testify to the return on investment for the institution, nursing mothers, and families. Seventy-one percent of respondents indicated that the program positively affected their work or academic performance to a *significant* degree. Fifty-five percent stated that without the support they would have taken increased vacation, sick, or leave time. One participant commented: "Our loyalty to UC Davis is much greater because of this and childcare on campus. The connections I have made at breastfeeding groups and daycare have also been beneficial for my work." Eighty-nine percent of respondents indicated that the Breastfeeding Support Program made it possible to work towards personal breastfeeding goals. Comments included: "It is pretty much the main reason why I breastfed my baby for 12 months." And, "I breastfed both my children eight-plus months while working full time; this would not have been possible without the convenient pumping stations around campus." And, "The Breastfeeding Support Program provided better expertise than the local hospital where my baby arrived more than two months early and was in the NICU. Without having attended the group before his birth, I would have had much greater difficulty feeding him breastmilk which reduced his risk for life-threatening complications."

Centralized Administration Provides Economy of Scale and Integrated Services

The UC Davis Breastfeeding Support Program has been centrally administered since it began. Originally, responsibility for the program was an assigned duty of the Child Care Coordinator position. Today it is part of the University's robust WorkLife portfolio. The administrative components encompass:

- Development, implementation, and management of infrastructure, services, and facilities;
- Budget planning and financial management;
- Marketing;
- Evaluation and process improvement;
- Policy and compliance;
- Campus and community liaison.

An online registration system facilitates data collection and connects participants to the program's lactation consultant, a directory of sites, and resource and referral assistance for childcare and other family services.

Formal evaluations were conducted annually for the first decade. Feedback is now gained through ongoing communication with program participants and stakeholders, and periodic surveys.

Breastfeeding Helps UC Davis Be Green

Sustainability is a core campus value. In 2012, *Sierra* magazine named UC Davis the nation's "Coolest School" for its sustainability initiatives and climate change efforts in the areas of transportation, lighting, recycling, and green purchasing. Lo and behold, breastfeeding is a sustainable practice, too. The American Academy of Pediatrics states that "breastfeeding is lean, green, and clean...it saves water and it doesn't use energy for manufacturing or pollute the environment with garbage or manufacturing air pollution" (American Academy of Pediatrics, 2012).

Beware, however, that the reduce-reuse-recycle mantra is not advisable for portable breast pumps. The Food and Drug Administration and La Leche League International address the risks of re-using "open system" pumps (Mohrbacher, 2004). Faced with the question, the campus sustainability planner, a former participant of the UC Davis Breastfeeding Support Program, has teamed with the lactation consultant to offer guidance on responsible disposal methods. Women who have weaned and inquire about donating their portable pumps and equipment for use by others are to take them to a household hazardous materials waste collection site.

BEST PRACTICE: In line with their campus values, UC Davis embraced the "lean, green, and clean" sustainable practice characteristic of breastfeeding and further considered the environmental impact of pump disposal in its approach to educating and informing breastfeeding women.

Two Decades of Service Lead to Better Breastfeeding Outcomes for UC Davis Nursing Mothers

When the UC Davis Breastfeeding Support Program was launched in 1995, it was very much a novel concept and pioneering effort, awkward to navigate at times, but well received and supported by the campus and local community. The program's founders hoped to do more than help women achieve their breastfeeding goals. They also aimed to change cultural views of breastfeeding and set an example for other workplaces and academic institutions. Mission accomplished.

References

American Academy of Pediatrics. (2012, March 1). Policy Statement: Breastfeeding and the use of human milk. *Pediatrics 129*(3), e827-e841. doi: 10.1542/peds.2011-3552.

Mason, M. (2009). Better educating our new breadwinners: Creating opportunities for all women to succeed in the workforce. In Boushey, H. & O'Leary, A. (Eds.), The Shriver Report: A woman's nation changes everything. (pp. 160-193). Washington, DC: Center for American Progress.

Mohrbacher, N. (2004, June/July). Are used breast pumps a good option? Issues to consider. *Leaven, 40*(3), 54-55. Retrieved October 19, 2013 from http://www.llli.org/llleaderweb/lv/lvjunjul04p54.html

Chapter Five
The University of Arizona Life & Work Connections: Lactation Resources with a Life Cycle Approach

Caryn Jung, Jan Sturges, Darci Thompson

There is a growing body of research that affirms the health and wellness benefits of breastmilk for babies. Studies name stronger immune systems to counter against bacteria and viruses, nutrients designed to promote brain and physical development, and special opportunities for parent and child bonding (National Institutes of Health, 2013; U.S. Department of Health and Human Services, 2011).

Mothers' contributions to the nation's labor force and the composition of students enrolled in colleges and universities indicate the continued need for strategic lactation resources at work and school. The Bureau of Labor Statistics reports, "The labor force participation rate—the percent of the population working or looking for work—for all mothers with children under age 18 was 70.5 percent in 2012" (U.S. Department of Labor, 2012). Since 1988, the number of females in post-baccalaureate programs has exceeded the number of males (U.S. Department of Education, 2012).

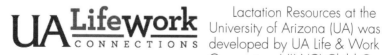

Figure 5.1

Lactation Resources at the University of Arizona (UA) was developed by UA Life & Work Connections' (LWC) Child Care and Family Resources Program (CCFR) to support employee and student parents, so mothers and babies could continue to reap the health benefits that breastmilk provides (Figure 5.1). Lactation Resources assists families with complementary strategies regarding an effective return to work, life, and classroom commitments.

To offer the reader with context, "the mission of the University of Arizona is to provide a comprehensive, high-quality education that engages our students in discovery through research and broad-based scholarship." Established in 1885, UA is the state's land-grant university and is ranked #19 among all public universities by the National Science Foundation as a premier research university. The University offers undergraduate and graduate degrees from 20 colleges and 11 schools on three campuses, which include Tucson's main campus, with a health sciences center and teaching hospital, the Phoenix College of Medicine and health sciences campus, and a campus in Sierra Vista. With additional research park, cooperative extension, and other settings, the UA reaches every Arizona county and five tribal reservations. Over 15,000 individuals teach and serve at the University of Arizona, on behalf of more than 37,000 undergraduate, graduate, and professional and medical students (University of Arizona, 2013b).

This chapter identifies how LWC's programs, services, and life cycle approach served as a foundation for the design, creation, implementation, and management of Lactation Resources at the University of Arizona. The authors also highlight the importance of developing and maintaining campus collaborations that support its continued success.

UA Life & Work Connections: An Integrated Program Model

LWC is the University's designated work-life office. The program provides consultation, information, and resources to its campus community (faculty, staff, and students) with seamless access to master's level professionals that have diverse expertise and experience in the fields of early care and education, eldercare, gerontology, and work-life. This includes counsel regarding campus lactation resources, strategies on selecting care settings that support lactation needs, and access to campus lactation spaces that facilitate individual wellbeing for mom and baby. A guiding value for LWC is the principle of complementary life and work development:

> "As life offers predictable milestones—birth, growing up, education, relationships, family, aging—work has its own progression: choosing a career, starting a job, training, developing competence, advancement, and the transition into retirement. Life & Work Connections provides life cycle services to complement the work cycles of UA employees and students…" (University of Arizona, 2013a).

By promoting healthy lifestyles and balance in work and life endeavors, employees and students can maximize their potential at work and in the classroom, as well as foster meaningful engagement in their personal lives. LWC's programs design and deliver value-added whole-person health services, educational programs, and comprehensive web-based resources in the following areas:

- **Childcare and Family Resources** – CCFR. Customized childcare consultations and referrals, lactation consultations and resources, a subsidized sick child and emergency/back-up care program, financial assistance for qualifying childcare costs, presentations.

- **Eldercare and Life Cycle Resources** – ECLCR. Personalized local and long distance resources and referrals, online caregiving tools, caregiver resource guide, presentations.

- **Employee Assistance Counseling/Consultation** – EACC. Individual counseling and consultations on work and personal issues, presentations.

- **Employee Wellness and Health Promotion** – EWHP. Nutrition and fitness counseling, health screenings, special events, presentations.

- **Work/Life Support** – WLS. Consultations on work-life issues and proposal strategies using the University's "Flexible Work Arrangements Guide," presentations.

These programs support the campus community with five specialized services. As individual issues are identified, LWC's multidisciplinary program structure and practice permits the staff to anticipate increasingly complex and multi-generational employee and student needs. This includes the ability to refer individuals to other professionals within the department that can help them address a continuum of life cycle circumstances. The depth and flexibility of this model supports a resilient and agile university in meeting its local, national, and global commitments.

BEST PRACTICE: At UA overall employee and student wellbeing, including lactation resources for mothers and babies, is supported through institutional leadership and vision promoting the critical infrastructure necessary to develop, expand, and sustain Life & Work Connections' integrated, holistic, and multidisciplinary programs and practices with a life-cycle approach.

Effective UA Campus Planning, Development, and Implementation

Time, space, support, and education about the benefits of breastfeeding are four critical elements needed for fostering an employee or student's ability to successfully combine campus life and

95

breastfeeding. When these individuals believe that they are better parents *and* better workers or students because of their positive experience with campus and worksite lactation resources, they communicate their successes with colleagues, family, and friends. Their personal stories promote community-wide understanding about the value of lactation resources and support, and validate that these aforementioned factors are necessary for the success of an employee and student lactation program (U.S. Breastfeeding Committee, 2010). This premise is underscored by one student and mother who described to the LWC CCFR Specialist how important it was for her to have accessible parking close to her classes so that she could leave campus to provide breastmilk for her baby at a nearby early care and education program, and return in time to attend her next class without being late or missing it altogether. The CCFR Specialist consulted with other campus partners, and arrangements were made to accommodate the student so that she could fulfill her responsibilities both as a mother and as a student (Figure 5.2).

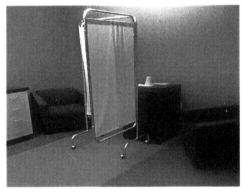

Figure 5.2 Lactation Room Set Up Using a Divider

In another example, LWC collaborations (based on insights from medical college leaders) resulted in the establishment of a dedicated lactation room (Figure 5.3). In this case, once again, a student indicated that

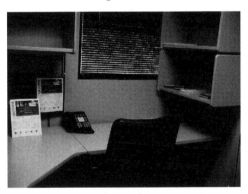

Figure 5.3 Dedicated Lactation Room

the accessibility of a lactation room on campus afforded her greater opportunities for both on-site studying and medical library access, as well as the opportunity to provide breastmilk for her child.

BEST PRACTICE: UA considered broader implications of advocating for and addressing student needs, not only employee needs, which may apply to visitors, too.

LWC began promoting the health, recruitment, and retention benefits of lactation in one-on-one consultations with employee and student mothers, in departmental presentations, orientations and workshops, and in campus and web-based communications. The information gathered from these discussions was included in a subsidy grant proposal that culminated in funding for LWC's *Mommy Connections* program, discussed later in the chapter. As part of this pilot program, lactation subsidies were developed to promote breastfeeding opportunities for women who may not have otherwise considered breastmilk for their babies due to associated costs, no prior experience as a mother, or lack of familiarity with these options.

While these strategies for developing Lactation Resources were in progress, LWC evaluated feedback and emerging questions from employee and student expectant parents about the need for lactation assistance and private spaces. It was difficult to know whether intermittent inquiries reflected an accurate subset of returning employee and student mothers, or whether interest and need was greater than the number of requests. During this process, it became apparent that identifying a systemic approach would best serve the needs of employees, students, and the institution.

This systemic approach included an assessment of existing resources, such as partnerships with university committees, administrative colleagues, facilities, and delivery systems, and the capability of promoting and expanding lactation spaces over time to serve the potential growth of women who would benefit from a comprehensive lactation program. Once the necessary information had been gathered, LWC initiated discussions with the university's medical center and other important stakeholders, such as departments and colleges, employees, students, women's interests, student governance, cultural diversity, and other campus populations.

Increasing awareness and appreciation about lactation needs and resources occurred by fostering established and potential campus relationships, and emphasizing employer-supported and personal and public health benefits. Honoring personal, cultural, and other salient features within a campus system optimizes a family's healthy recovery and connection to University resources, such as infant childcare options that affirm lactation preferences. It was agreed that LWC's Child Care and Family Resources professionals would be a good conduit for educating and engaging UA faculty, staff, and students about lactation resources and consultations from a psychosocial perspective. This supports personal wellbeing and an effective and well-prepared transition for returning to work or class.

There was also agreement that the medical center should continue to provide medically based lactation counseling by healthcare professionals to mothers during pregnancy and/or through the postpartum period, which would include information about the benefits of mothers' breastmilk for babies and rental of breastfeeding equipment. In a clinical setting, healthcare colleagues assist mothers, babies, and families with a healthy recuperation and an understanding of how to navigate healthcare options that support an effective and well-prepared transition to new routines at home following the birth of a baby. This complementary consultative partnership achieved the objectives necessary to provide new mothers with access to information about healthy breastfeeding practices (according to the standards of the International Lactation Consultant Association), and strengthened campus-wide alliances, which evolved into collaborations for implementing a broader range of educational opportunities and lactation spaces for Lactation Resources.

> BEST PRACTICE: Partnering with UA medical center helped to develop and sustain optimal lactation practices and address complex needs of mother, baby, and family wellbeing, as well as classroom and manager responsibilities.

The relationships developed through these discussions provided a richer foundation for LWC's subsequent lactation subsidy and enhanced consultation program, *Mommy Connections* (outlined below). One additional outcome of these discussions was a recommendation to fund and create centrally located lactation space within the Arizona Student Unions system. The success of this initiative led to a space being allocated at an affiliate Arizona Student Union's site located on another part of campus. The steady growth and progression of Lactation Resources became a model for other universities as a noteworthy recruitment and retention practice.

Today, the 2010 Patient Protection and Affordable Care Act requires expanded coverage for breastfeeding assistance and counseling, access to breastfeeding supplies for pregnant and nursing women, and uniform standards regarding adequate break times for nursing mothers. UA's growing Lactation Resources and *Mommy Connections*, along with the planning and implementation efforts regarding ACA compliance, guided the institution's best practice standards. They include a plan of support by department heads for individual employee mothers who are breastfeeding, provisions for a private location (not a restroom) to express breastmilk, and a reasonable amount of break time to accommodate this process for up to one year after the birth of a child.

Designing a Multi-Site Network of Campus Lactation Spaces

A challenge and opportunity for promoting lactation resources and education, and systemic space expansion at the University of Arizona is its broad presence throughout the state. A heightened visibility of available Tucson campus lactation spaces (such as at centrally located buildings) ultimately underscored the need for more options within the main campus, with the goal of continued progress at other UA sites. The CCFR Specialist elicited input from employee and student mothers about their lactation needs, as well as privacy concerns. Informal queries ranged from solicited feedback to follow-up communications. LWC researched and reviewed requests from mothers about lactation resources, utilization, and their satisfaction. In general, mothers used designated lactation spaces whenever available. Furthermore, employee lactation examples included the use of one's office or a colleague's vacated office space during coordinated break and lunch times. For students, this included access to a private room with assistance from their professors or department.

This information was helpful in determining how to develop and implement additional lactation spaces that were readily accessible. It also provided valuable data for recommending increases in lactation funding, spaces, and education. LWC's continuing dialogue regarding permissible lactation areas within ACA guidelines helped the CCFR Specialist identify appropriate alternatives for a space thought to be satisfactory. Based on complementary childcare and lactation consultations, convenient breastfeeding options in the returning mothers' work buildings were established, benefiting both current and future mothers.

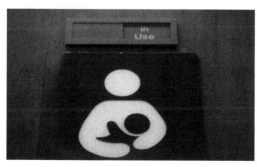

Figure 5.4 International Breastfeeding Symbol on Lactation Room Door

Awareness and use of lactation rooms originated from informal sharing amongst mothers, collegial relationships through *Mommy Connections* and other University affiliations, and from individual and departmental requests for assistance in establishing new lactation areas. Developing the initial network of lactation locations at the University was a grassroots, collaborative effort, which, in turn, served as a catalyst for increased institutional planning and partnerships.

To extend support at its many campus locations, the CCFR Specialist facilitated student, faculty, employee, and supervisor understanding about lactation needs with suggested strategies and guidelines that reflected local adaptability and 24/7 access. Promoting ideas on how to establish lactation spaces, organizational and commercial lactation resources, and the availability of the International Breastfeeding Symbol were also initiated by Lactation Resources (Figure 5.4).

> BEST PRACTICE: Providing 24/7 access to lactation support increases access and availability for UA students and employees working second and third shifts.

From a future planning perspective, LWC now complements the expertise provided by the University's Planning, Design & Construction staff with information from organizations that have already developed lactation room design specifications, such as the American Institute of Architects. They include design standards, specifications, and requirements for new construction, as well as

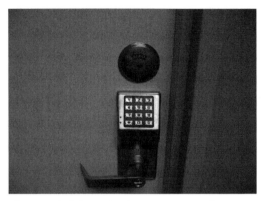

Figure 5.5 Door Lock on Lactation Room – Allows Moms to Access Room Without a Key

retrofitting existing buildings (Figure 5.5). These discussions have led to creative planning for new lactation spaces and modifications for existing ones, along with preferences for allowing timely access between buildings as lactation sites develop throughout campus. This has given Lactation Resources planners the opportunity to discuss UA's compliance with the 2010 Affordable Care Act standards. Future plans include promoting this partnership and policy with formal communications throughout the campus community and within the fields of higher education and work-life.

> BEST PRACTICE: A formal UA lactation space policy for new construction and retrofitting of locations in existing buildings is part of a systemic model for increasing the number of lactation spaces on campus.

Managing the University of Arizona's Lactation Resources is a complex, detailed, and iterative process. Oversight requires knowledge of maternal and pediatric health research, policy and statute information, space design and development issues, fiscal, academic, and calendar year schedules, lactation supplies and equipment elements speak to the extensive range of knowledge required to nurture such initiatives in a campus environment. Another valuable complement of this integrated model is the collaborative partnering, acumen, and interdisciplinary agility of LWC's master's level staff, who serve people across the life span.

> BEST PRACTICE: Strategic partnering can enhance competencies and resources needed to address lactation-related inquiries ranging from health research, policy, statute, and facilities issues to campus systems and populations, lactation resources, and compliance standards.

Serving UA individuals and sites across the state of Arizona, LWC is strongly committed to assisting employee and student mothers who wish to provide breastmilk for their babies. In collaboration with university colleagues, we continue to initiate, promote, and complement efforts that support child, individual, and family wellbeing. Key to this collaboration is the leadership of colleges and departments who are dedicated to promoting Lactation Resources by establishing and maintaining their respective lactation spaces, accepting LWC's invitation to recommend these sites on campus, and supporting universal best practices and ACA standards.

Mommy Connections: The Evolution of a University of Arizona Campus and Medical Center Collaboration

Before the nation's 2010 Affordable Care Act, LWC's *Mommy Connections* was a subsidy program, which provided lactating mothers with a reduction in the first month's rental cost or purchase price of a breast pump. *Mommy Connections* also facilitated mothers' access to clinical, lactation counseling support, with the goal of enhancing their personal and campus experiences through comprehensive LWC and hospital assistance. Mothers are now referred to their healthcare providers for advice about rental choices, according to ACA standards, and the feasibility of purchasing breast pumps from their respective insurance carriers.

In tandem with *Mommy Connections*, UA Human Resources affirmed a policy that supports breastfeeding mothers by allowing them a reasonable amount of break time at work for using a breast pump in appropriate and comfortable spaces. It states, "Employees who are nursing are provided with reasonable unpaid break time to express breastmilk after the birth of the child, as long as providing such a break does not unduly disrupt operations. The department head will make reasonable efforts to provide the employee a private location, not a breastmilk after the birth of the child, as long as providing such a break does not unduly disrupt operations. The department head will make reasonable efforts to provide the employee a private location, not a restroom, for nursing and/or expressing breastmilk. The regulation requires availability of the break time for one year after the child's birth, and department heads are encouraged to be flexible when developing a plan of support for an individual employee" (University of Arizona, 2013c).

No longer a pilot project, *Mommy Connections* continues to evolve regarding features that support ACA standards and hospital needs, and contributes to sustainable and effective campus work-life practices. Childcare and campus lactation room referrals for employees and students that are made by the medical center to LWC, as well as referrals made by LWC to the hospital regarding mother and baby lactation inquiries, are a continuing facet of *Mommy Connections'* original intent and practice concerning access and education. The *Mommy Connections* partnership demonstrates unique and responsive assistance to employee and student mothers and their babies during a very personal and important time in their work and life experiences by upholding health practices and collaborations with stakeholders as part of a broader campus enterprise.

Higher education and healthcare settings can routinely experience administrative, organizational, and other changes that influence the delivery of services. Agility within LWC's Lactation Resources provides the foundation from which to modify and model the broadest range of campus community options available at

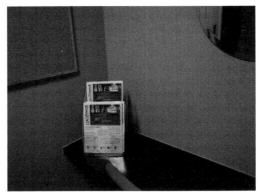

Figure 5.6 Lactation Room Brochures

any given time. The CCFR Specialist continues to work with campus committees and interested departments on the development of lactation spaces. LWC facilitates referrals to a board certified and registered lactation consultant as needed for personalized consultations. Educational resources, lactation guidelines, frequently asked questions about breastfeeding and a family-friendly brochure with lactation and childcare resources are also disseminated to faculty, staff, and students at the University through various modalities: listservs, UA publications, website, and social media (Figure 5.6).

In particular, the University of Arizona has been identified as providing a best practice work-life program website in higher education based on a research project conducted by the College and University Work-Life-Family Association and Alfred P. Sloan Foundation. A key project focus involved: "...identifying best practices in site layout, design, and content from campuses across the nation. Data was collected and analyzed from 340 higher education and work-life websites, including those of all CUWFA members" (CUWFA, 2013). The University was lauded for its comprehensive suite of work-life services, including LWC's Lactation Resources, and the ability to effectively communicate and promote these services on the web. Current and former work-life best practices commendations about the University of Arizona, encompassing lactation and other resources, include recognition as a leadership model among public, private, and higher education settings (University of Arizona, 2013a).

> BEST PRACTICE: Affiliations with organizations that value lactation support programs and other work-life efforts can help universities develop best practices.

LWC continues to support individuals, the institution, and well-regarded health practices as part of a broader campus enterprise with its medical center relationships. This commitment includes cross-referrals to other LWC professionals as appropriate, facilitating the development of lactation spaces, sharing implementation strategies and educational resources, and providing access to a board certified and registered lactation consultant for personalized consultations. Examples of positive feedback about Lactation Resources include the following:

- "As a mom, a public health professional, and a proud employee in the [UA] Wildcat family, I believe the benefits of breastfeeding are countless. The support from UA Life & Work Connections was essential to my success in balancing life, work, and providing breastmilk to my young son..." (Public health professional).

- "Promoting optimal beginnings for new mothers and their babies is a shared value between UA Life & Work Connections and lactation services at the University's medical center. Supporting employee and student parents with the important transition back to campus continues to be an enriching experience on many levels. It is rewarding to know that our collegial example strengthens the work and life foundation families seek towards a healthy start for children" (Medical center professional).

Conclusion and Recommendations

Steps and ideas to establish and foster lactation resources in higher education and in other workplace settings include:

- Conducting thoughtful research and preparation for developing or strengthening an effective lactation practice model.

- Identifying key campus stakeholders, partnerships, and collaborative efforts.

- Evaluating campus resources—physical location and architectural design requirements, compliance with ACA policies and standards, funding sources.

- Fostering institutional commitment for integrated and sustainable program services.

- Promoting lactation as an investment, not an expense. (According to the U.S. Breastfeeding Committee, 2010, lactation resources in the workplace generate a cost savings of $3 for every $1 invested in breastfeeding support.)

- Publicizing lactation resources through available media.

Lactation Resources through Life & Work Connections at the University of Arizona demonstrates that a multi-site university environment can be a progressive place to work and learn when administrators, staff, and departments partner with work-life professionals to develop and implement programs that balance best practices from a business perspective with the best interests of their constituents. According to one College of Management colleague, "As a University of Arizona faculty member and working mother, I can state that the very personal experiences of faculty, staff, and students coupled with the university's efforts to maintain its business and management objectives are compelling reasons to provide lactation assistance. Life & Work Connections offers a leadership model that promotes employee recruitment and retention in the context of organizational best practices" (C. Gilland, personal communication, January 28, 2013).

References

College and University Work-Life-Family Association (CUWFA). (2013). Retrieved July 3, 2103 from http://www.cuwfa.org/toolkit-public.

National Institutes of Health. (2013). Medline Plus. "Breastfeeding." U.S. National Library of Medicine. 8600 Rockville Pike, Bethesda, MD. 20894. Retrieved January 16, 2013 from http://www.nlm.nih.gov/medlineplus/breastfeeding. html.

U.S. Breastfeeding Committee. "Workplace Accommodations to Support and Protect Breastfeeding." Washington, DC: U.S. Breastfeeding Committee; 2010. P.9. Retrieved February 6, 2013 from http://www.usbreastfeeding. org/LinkClick.aspx?link=Publications%2fWorkplace-Background-2010-USBC. pdf&tabid=70&mid=388.

U.S. Department of Education, National Center for Education Statistics. (2012). *Digest of Education Statistics, 2011* Chapter 3. Retrieved February 1, 2013 from http://nces.ed.gov/programs/digest/d11/ch_3.aspp.

U.S. Department of Health and Human Services Office of Women's Health. (2011). "Your Guide to Breastfeeding." Retrieved from http://www.womenshealth. gov/publications/our-publications/breastfeeding-guide/breastfeedingguide-general-english.pdf.

U.S. Department of Labor, Bureau of Labor Statistics. Employment Characteristics of Families – 2012. Retrieved August 22, 2013 from http://www.bls.gov/news. release/pdf/famee.pdf.

University of Arizona. (2013a). "Philosophy & mission." Retrieved July 3, 2013 from http://lifework.arizona.edu/wwa/philosophy.

University of Arizona. (2013b). "Fact Book at a Glance - Quick Reference 2011-2012." Retrieved July 3, 2013 from http://factbook.arizona.edu/2011-12/ at_a_glance.

University of Arizona. (2013c). "Lactation Resources." Retrieved July 3, 2013 from http://lifework.arizona.edu/cc/lactation_information

Chapter Six
Back to Work and Breastfeeding at Michigan State University: It's Just Good Sense

Lori Strom

Michigan State University (MSU) was founded in 1855 in East Lansing, Michigan, as the nation's pioneer land-grant university and was a prototype for 69 other land-grant institutions under the Morrill Act of 1862. Currently, MSU enrolls nearly 50,000 students and employs approximately 5,000 faculty and academic staff and 6,400 support staff. Fifty-two percent of the students, 33% of faculty (academic and administrative), and 63% of the support staff are women.

The main campus is large, with 5,200 acres of land and 532 buildings, which creates a challenge to establish breastfeeding rooms across campus. Yet MSU is committed to providing a work and educational environment that supports students and employees' professional and personal lives. MSU's administration understands that by creating an inclusive campus community, while supporting breastfeeding students, staff, and faculty, it can cultivate, recruit, and retain a world-class workforce and student body.

The University continues the land-grant mission to provide quality educational opportunities to vulnerable populations of the state of Michigan, as well as conducting global research as a Tier I research institution. To fulfill the land-grant mission, the University provides community outreach to residents of the state of Michigan (through the 83 MSU County Extension offices), as well as the greater Lansing area. Through the MSU Extension offices across the state, breastfeeding support and research initiatives reach into the community off campus. MSU also participates in community initiatives, such as the Capital Area Breastfeeding Coalition, that positively impact breastfeeding mothers and promote a supportive environment for any breastfeeding women who are on campus and need to feed their babies or pump their breastmilk.

"Bolder by Design; Working Together. Getting it Done."

Community collaboration is a cornerstone of the MSU success story. In 2005, President Lou Anna K. Simon launched the strategic imperative "Bolder by Design," highlighting five areas in which MSU must excel and innovate to fulfill its commitment to transformation and to become the model land-grant university for the 21st century:

1. Enhance the student experience;
2. Enrich community, economic, and family life;
3. Expand international reach;
4. Increase research opportunities;
5. Strengthen stewardship.

As one of the strategic imperatives emphasizes "Enrich community, economic, and family life," the University is well poised to support the needs of breastfeeding mothers and their babies.

Past Institutional Initiatives Support Women and Build a Solid Foundation

In the 1970s, issues pertaining to women were addressed by the administration. In an effort to reach women across campus from all three constituent groups—faculty, staff, and students—three women's advisory committees were created to represent each group, reporting to their respective leaders. Over forty years later, all three groups continue to meet regularly. Since the 1980s, MSU has informally provided flexible work opportunities and private spaces for nursing mothers. Individual requests were met in a decentralized manner in certain departments and buildings, but no formal policies were established.

All three of these women's advisory committees have addressed breastfeeding support concerns at some point over the past four decades. However, most recently a unique breastfeeding initiative was created that makes MSU stand out as an exemplary and supportive institution of higher education.

In 1999 in response to "support staff women" requests for breastfeeding rooms, a formal recommendation was made to the administration to institutionalize support for breastfeeding mothers. In response to their request, a memo was sent to departments across campus to encourage supervisors to be supportive of mothers returning from maternity leave. Managers were encouraged to provide nursing mothers with a private space to feed and/or pump and a flexible work schedule to make time available to pump as needed. However, this response did not include a directive to establish rooms.

During this time when the administration was encouraging a supportive work environment, there were only a few unofficial, designated breastfeeding rooms on campus that were primarily set up by departments, and not established by the administration. Frequently, mothers working in various departments across campus took it upon themselves to create rooms in their buildings. They used existing rooms, such as women's lounges, kitchenettes, and break rooms, as their designated "unofficial" breastfeeding rooms. Many were informal; others were sanctioned by the department administrator. "Breastfeeding room" signs were displayed on some doors.

A Collaboration of "Like-Minded" Professionals Moves the Breastfeeding Agenda Forward

The MSU Family Resource Center was established in 1994 to address childcare issues on campus in response to a campus-wide survey of faculty, staff, and student families' childcare needs. The Family Resource Center is a small two-person office housed in Human Resources and is funded by Student Affairs and Services. Over the past 20 years, the Family Resource Center mission has expanded to support the dependent care and work-life needs of students, staff, and faculty with a lifespan approach from pregnancy to eldercare.

In response to employees that were requesting breastfeeding support and designated pumping rooms in the late 1990s, the MSU Family Resource Center convened a multifaceted stakeholder group of campus representatives to become the Breastfeeding Support Advisory Committee, an informal, ad-hoc committee. Their first meeting was held in the beginning of 2000. The institution-wide message from the Breastfeeding Support Advisory Committee was to promote the benefits of breastfeeding support, which could reduce absenteeism and healthcare costs, and enhance the health of the mothers and their babies, improve morale and job satisfaction, and improve loyalty and commitment to MSU.

BEST PRACTICE: A strength of the Breastfeeding Support Advisory Committee at MSU was in its diverse membership, which included nursing mothers, student parents, staff and faculty, lactation consultants, nurses, doctors, and childcare providers.

The goals of the Breastfeeding Support Advisory Committee were to help promote options for mothers returning to work after maternity leave and to support their continuation of breastfeeding. The committee helped to promote a campus-wide initiative to encourage supervisors to allow flexibility in the schedules of nursing mothers who need time and space to nurse or express/pump breastmilk during the workday. The Breastfeeding Support Advisory Committee advocated for specific employer policies to encourage the MSU administration and supervisors to support breastfeeding mothers.

BEST PRACTICE: The Breastfeeding Support Advisory Committee's decision to focus its communication on the impact breastfeeding has on business-specific indicators, such as reduced absenteeism and healthcare costs, and increased job satisfaction and productivity, provided a buy-in platform for lactation support at MSU.

The Breastfeeding Support Advisory Committee met regularly until late 2001. Their primary accomplishments included enhanced publicity that brought more awareness of breastfeeding issues and needs across campus. They created a breastfeeding support brochure that was designed for student, staff, and faculty mothers and their supervisors that continues to be disseminated through the Family Resource Center. Additionally, they established a lunch and learn program for expectant parents that centered on breastfeeding and an email listserv for MSU breastfeeding moms. As a collaborative venture between the Breastfeeding Support Advisory Committee and Health 4U, the MSU Health and Wellness program led by the MSU University Physician's office started a breastfeeding education series in 2000. These free learn-at-lunch classes have been offered to approximately 300 hundred MSU students, staff, and faculty, and their spouses/partners every fall and spring semester for almost 14 years.

BEST PRACTICE: MSU included clinical support and expertise in its implementation of their lactation program for working mothers.

During each fall and spring semester, a lactation consultant leads the series, which includes the following sessions: *An introduction to breastfeeding* – explaining the benefits of breastfeeding; *The baby is here! How to get started* – describing the mechanics of breastfeeding with positioning, latching-on, feeding patterns, and challenges; *Maintaining breastfeeding* – considering Mom's lifestyle with tips on expressing and storing milk and returning to work and pumping; and

Breastfeeding transitions – preparing to end breastfeeding, introducing solid foods, and weaning. During the last class session of the series, a drawing is held for one of the class participants to win a copy of the classic book by La Leche League, *"The Womanly Art of Breastfeeding."* The feedback on the class series has been very positive, and many mothers who participated in the classes together have remained friends since their children are the same age.

The last initiative of the committee was the establishment of an electronic breastfeeding email listserv. In an effort to connect breastfeeding moms and to have an opportunity to disseminate information pertaining to the common interests of breastfeeding mothers across campus and in the community, the breastfeeding email listserv was set up for MSU staff, faculty, students, and local professionals. Currently, 150 mothers are members of the email listserv.

Inventory of Informal Breastfeeding Spaces Leads to Master List of Rooms

The first campus-wide inventory of space to establish breastfeeding rooms was completed in 2001. The Family Resource Center designed a survey that was mailed to "building contacts" in approximately 1,044 units across campus in more than 500 buildings. Subsequent surveys were sent in 2004 and 2007 with similar results.

Of the more than 1,000 questionnaires that were mailed, 143 surveys were returned. The 14% response rate can be attributed to the fact that the survey came from a support service office, the Family Resource Center, and response was not mandated by executive management. The takeaway lesson is that a survey may yield a higher percent of respondents when it is sent from high-level authorities, with federal law to back it up (as was the case in 2010 with the ACA mandate of established breastfeeding rooms in workplaces of more than 50 employees).

Of the 143 respondents to the first survey sent to MSU units by the Family Resource Center, 30 reported they had no space available for nursing mothers to use. Of the 143 replies, 44 reported that they had designated rooms, would work with the individual, or had potential space moms could use. The other 69 units did not comment on their space availability. At this time, there was no institutionalized building standard to establish breastfeeding rooms on campus, and there was no public listing available to mothers looking for an appropriate pumping room in their buildings. Yet, because of the informal building surveys conducted in 2001, 2004, and 2007, the Family Resource Center had a list of buildings/rooms they could refer to when a mother called looking for an appropriate breastfeeding space in her building. Family Resource Center staff could give them a contact person's name and information, and a possible room number that they could use, but the lists could not be made public, as the administration had not endorsed the rooms for publication. These surveys laid a strong foundation for the design of the Google Map (described below) that was established in 2011.

BEST PRACTICE: MSU conducted a formal environmental scan to assess the inventory of space in the beginning of their plan.

Creating an Agenda for Breastfeeding at MSU

Despite supportive evidence from The American Academy of Pediatrics (2005) and the Business Case for Breastfeeding, many infants are not receiving breastmilk as recommended. Michigan mothers initiate and continue breastfeeding at rates below the national average. According to the Michigan Council for Maternal and Child Health, Medicaid Breastfeeding Policy Brief in 2011, the State of Michigan got a "D" on the breastfeeding report card from the Centers for Disease Control and Prevention. As one of the largest employers in mid-Michigan, MSU has an impact on the health and wellbeing of thousands of mothers and their babies. As a tireless advocate for breastfeeding support at MSU, the Family Resource Center Coordinator attended the U.S. Department of Health and Human Services, Health Resource and Service Administration's Maternal and Child Health Bureau and the Office on Women's Health two-day conference, *"Implementing the Business Case for Breastfeeding in Your Community"* in 2009, which provided insight into strategies to reduce the social, structural, and environmental barriers to breastfeeding that mothers encounter, so that MSU moms can continue breastfeeding after returning from maternity leave. The evidence presented reinforced the need, as well as the institutional and employee personal benefits for MSU as an employer.

Approach Backed by Breastfeeding Research

Two faculty at MSU, along with their colleagues from the University of South Carolina, used focus groups to examine the perspectives of managers and employees toward workplace breastfeeding support in a variety of settings throughout the State of Michigan (Chow, Smithey Fulmer & Olson, 2011). The results indicated that managers' attitudes influence female employees' perceptions of workplace breastfeeding support. Eventually, results of this study will be useful for developing an instrument to measure MSU managers' attitudes toward supporting breastfeeding.

In the meantime, informal assessments of mothers' needs for space to pump breastmilk were performed to establish a formalized approach to meeting their needs. The results of the informal campus surveys indicate that employees' perceptions of their managers' attitudes impacted women's comfort with pumping at their campus jobs.

In 2010, the informal survey was sent to 140 mothers on the MSU breastfeeding email listserv. Ninety-eight (70%) of the mothers replied, and their results indicated that on any given day approximately 100 student, staff, and faculty mothers were breastfeeding and needed a place to pump on campus.

Nearly 83% of moms indicated they breastfed in the past year, and 63% planned to breastfeed in the following year, with 85% of these women expecting to express/pump/feed in the workplace. Additionally, some of their comments in the open narrative section illustrated that mothers were more likely to pump if they had a private space and a supportive supervisor. They indicated they were often afraid to ask supervisors for support, flex time, and a private room:

- "I was actually too embarrassed to ask, so I would just run home and pump. It was a pain in the butt though. I wish I had a place at work that was private to do this."
- "I pumped in my car or drove home."
- "I have my own office with a door that locks. I was able to set up my pump, put a note on the door to not disturb, and pump in private."
- "I can lock myself in a conference room for privacy."

These responses back-up the research findings that mothers are often afraid to ask their supervisors for space to pump.

> BEST PRACTICE: MSU provides campus faculty with opportunities to conduct formal research that may inform current and/or future program components.

Paving the Road for the MSU Google Map of Nursing Mothers' Rooms; the Affordable Care Act

Following this survey and as a result of the ACA, which mandated employers with 50 or more employees to provide a private space and flexible work schedule to be able to pump up to the baby's first birthday, a formal approach to establishing rooms occurred at MSU. With the passage of the 2010 Affordable Care Act and Section 7 of the Fair Labor Standards Act, the Michigan State University administration requested major administrative units to identify rooms for nursing mothers. A memo was sent to deans, directors, and chairs from the Office for Inclusion and Intercultural Initiatives, Human Resources, and the Provost's office informing them about the passage of the new law and the need to establish locations that would be a functional space for expressing milk.

The memo continued, "the location does not have to be permanent but must be created and made available when needed and must be shielded from view and free from the possibility of intrusion by co-workers and the public. Restrooms, even if private, are not considered permissible locations."

The memo clarified the amendment applies to non-exempt (i.e., overtime eligible) employees for one year following birth, and requires the employer to provide a reasonable amount of break time to express milk "as frequently as needed by the nursing mother," noting that the time will vary depending on the individual.

One year later, another memo was sent to major administrative unit facility representatives from the Office of Planning and Budgets/Facilities Planning and Space Management to request the identification of rooms in buildings on and off campus, which would be available to nursing mothers. It was emphasized that the request was being made to ensure compliance with the ACA and was consistent with the University's effort to provide a supportive work environment for new mothers returning to work or school. The memo clarified the minimum requirements for the rooms:

- 4' x 5' private space (minimum);
- Lockable door;
- Chair and table;
- Electric outlet;

- Access to a sink (nearby in a restroom, break room, kitchenette);
- Adequate lighting.

Once the units responded to the request, a spreadsheet was created and approximately 88 rooms in more than 60 buildings were identified. The vision was to establish a room in every building with over 500 buildings on campus. But in the meantime, a clever Google map was created to give nursing mothers online access to private rooms in the buildings in which they work and go to class.

The Google map also lists the contact people, with their contact information, room hours, and numbers, and any other pertinent information to help women locate and identify appropriate spaces for their use. The Google Map was modeled after the "disability building access map" that was designed in the past to indicate buildings that have accessible entrances for wheelchairs. The MSU Geographic Information System Department created the electronic Google map of campus (Figure 6.1), which indicates all of the rooms and buildings with a "push pin" graphic.

> BEST PRACTICE: An interactive Google map was designed in 2010 to give nursing mothers easy access to more than 88 rooms in over 60 buildings with the formal establishment of designated private breastfeeding rooms across campus.

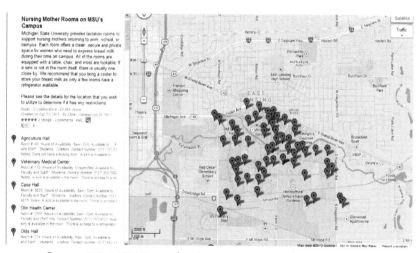

Figure 6.1 MSU Breastfeeding Room Google Map Image

Various web-based technologies exist that can be used to highlight and indicate the breastfeeding rooms on campus. The Google map was selected because it is the most accessible from all electronic devises. But because it is hard to maintain and update the data on the Google map, there is a future plan to switch technologies. It will be taken off the Google site and will be created on a new MSU system. The codes, written in-house, enable users to go from the spreadsheet to the map without problems and will ease future update and change processes. Further, the breastfeeding rooms are listed alphabetically.

Annual reminder notices are sent by the Office of Planning and Budgets to major administrative unit facility representatives and departments to be sure the room list is updated. Updates will occur periodically and will be communicated cooperatively between the units. The Family Resource Center also sends periodic updates, as mothers try to access rooms that may have been taken offline.

Essential Elements of MSU's Success Story

Funding for Breastfeeding Spaces

MSU construction standards include language for new and renovated buildings for "Personal Health Rooms" for any space that is more than $20,000 in building or renovation costs. A breastfeeding room is considered a "Personal Health Room" and would be centrally funded if the expenses exceeded $20,000. (A Personal Health Room is a quiet, private space where an employee may rest with a migraine headache, use insulin, or use for other personal needs.) In most cases the funding of the breastfeeding room space is the responsibility of departments, unless the cost is too high and prohibitive. In that case the central administration will cover the cost.

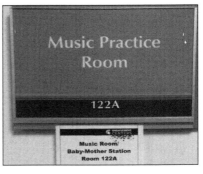

Figure 6.2a MSU Breastfeeding Room Sign

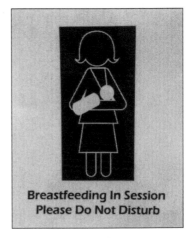

Figure 6.2b MSU Breastfeeding Room Sign

Managing Signage and Upkeep

In addition to the renovation costs, the departments are responsible for keeping the rooms clean and providing signage. Custodial staff clean the rooms as they do office space and

116

restrooms, and the departments unofficially designate a person to keep the rooms in order. The signage may be permanent or temporary, as needed for each use. There is no university signage standard for breastfeeding rooms because some of the rooms have multiple uses (i.e., conference rooms, lounges, and offices). Examples of signs include "Breastfeeding in Session; Please Do Not Disturb," "Private," "Breastfeeding Room," "Lactation Room," "Nursing Mother's Room," and the universal "Free to Feed" symbol (Figure 6.2 a, b, c).

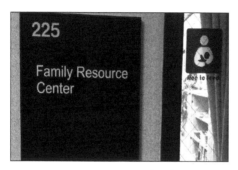

Figure 6.2c MSU Breastfeeding Room Sign

Providing Amenities

As previously mentioned, the minimum requirements for the rooms at MSU are basic. While other institutions may include hospital-grade breast pumps and attachment-kit supplies, mirrors, sinks, refrigerators, etc., MSU provides the space with access to a sink nearby and requires mothers to bring their own equipment for milk pumping and storage. Access to a refrigerator is preferred, but not required, as many mothers prefer to bring a portable cooler, rather than storing their milk in a public refrigerator (Figure 6.3).

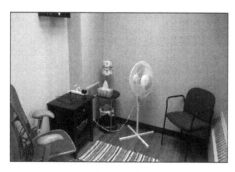

Figure 6.3 MSU Room

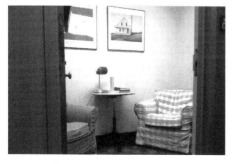

Figure 6.4 MSU Room

Identifying Campus Champions

Every institution of higher education needs a champion to shepherd community collaboration and breastfeeding support initiatives. The champions then need allies who are in a position of influence to help obtain buy-in from upper administrators and managers on campus.

Manager education and mentoring is imperative to create consistency of treatment across the institution. Knowledgeable and sensitive supervisors can ensure the success of nursing mothers to breastfeed their babies as long as possible, ideally up to one year of age. In large institutions such as MSU, you will find pockets of support, where some departments will be more supportive and breastfeeding friendly than others (Figure 6.4).

Annually, the Family Resource Center recognizes supervisors who are nominated by their employees because they are sensitive to and support the personal and family needs of their employees. The annual Outstanding Supervisor Award is held on National Bosses Day, October 16th, to award and celebrate the managers who support flexible work arrangements and their employees' personal needs, including breastfeeding mothers.

> BEST PRACTICE: Identifying and recognizing administrators and staff who support the program is a great way to build success, as demonstrated by MSU.

Creating Community Collaborations

Fulfilling its land-grant mission, the university provides community outreach to Michigan residents, as well as the greater Lansing area. An illustration of collaborative breastfeeding support is the relationship with the Capital Area Breastfeeding Coalition. The Capital Area Breastfeeding Coalition (CABC) is a team of breastfeeding professionals, lactation consultants, registered nurses, La Leche League leaders, and breastfeeding advocates in the Mid-Michigan/Lansing, Michigan area. This group formed to better serve and support breastfeeding mothers via education, advocacy, and resource support. Their goal is to increase the number and duration of women in the Lansing, Michigan area who initiate and continue exclusive breastfeeding through the recommended time period.

The CABC endorsed and advocated for the recent passage of a Breastfeeding Resolution for Ingham County, Michigan (where MSU resides). The resolution is a breastfeeding policy allowing women to breastfeed in any county building and makes public spaces "breastfeeding friendly." It was modeled after

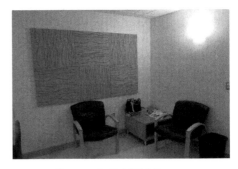

Figure 6.5 MSU Room

a Washtenaw County (Ann Arbor, Michigan) policy. The policy would mean staff at county-controlled properties, including courthouses, parks, and offices, could not discourage mothers from breastfeeding in public. As one of the largest employers in the capital region, MSU can serve as a workplace role model, in addition to providing academic and research support around breastfeeding (Figure 6.5).

When the Going Gets Tough, the Tough Get Going

Although it can be frustrating...the champions and advocates should never give up. For every advocacy effort made and every single room established, there is a mother who is able to continue breastfeeding her baby. And those who are in higher education know these things take time.

One of the biggest barriers to a successful breastfeeding support program is the communication of the resources to mothers and their supervisors. Communication of programs across a college campus can be challenging. Websites, brochures, email listservs, program directory listings, department meetings, educational class postings, and word of mouth are all common methods to get the word out about university breastfeeding support programs. The promotion needs to be ongoing; there will always be new mothers on campus that may be in need of these services.

Another challenge to be addressed involves maintaining a public listing of breastfeeding rooms (i.e., the MSU Google map). There is a need to keep the list current and up-to-date. When departments are overworked and overwhelmed with other important tasks, keeping breastfeeding support services and maps a priority can be difficult. If one unit is designated to be fully responsible for the program, it is more likely to be successful. Yet, at times, there is a need for multiple units to have responsibility in the promotion and room up-keep, which requires communication and collaboration between the units.

From a Work in Progress to a Work of Heart

The long history of breastfeeding support at MSU has been a "work in progress." For forty years the University has provided informal support in a decentralized manner in individual departments on a case-by-case basis. Currently, MSU provides space to support nursing mothers returning to work or school. Each room offers a clean, secure, and private space for women who need to express breastmilk during their time at MSU. All of the rooms are equipped with a table, chair, and are lockable. If a sink is not in the room itself, there is usually one close by. While many of the rooms have access to a refrigerator, we recommend that moms bring a cooler to store their breastmilk in the event that their location does not offer such access.

The ACA mandate led to the formalization of 88 breastfeeding rooms in 61 MSU buildings, which are currently illustrated with a unique Google map. However, additional rooms are still needed. Efforts at MSU to improve the workplace climate of breastfeeding support have a focus on formal programs and facilities, yet more mentoring of managers may provide knowledge of the benefits of breastfeeding support and improve supervisory practices toward breastfeeding mothers.

Since flexibility is a key component to successful breastfeeding for working women, resources have been developed and include a website with a self-guided workplace flexibility E-course for managers and employees, instructions for developing flexible work arrangements, a telecommuting guide, resource links, sample forms, and evaluation suggestions. Although MSU does not have a policy that mandates workplace flexibility, it is up to the supervisors' discretion if their employees can flex. The Flexible Work Arrangements Web page is located on the Human Resources Website, which gives it credibility for managers who are uncertain of their prerogative and the benefits of flexing schedules to accommodate nursing mothers.

Clearly, the implementation of the 2010 federal healthcare law (ACA) that mandates employers to support breastfeeding mothers with appropriate space and work place flexibility, propelled the MSU administration to formally request that the rooms be established in as many buildings as possible. As with Affirmative Action, FMLA, and ADA regulations, it is federal law that incentivizes workplace compliance.

MSU effectively has engaged champions across campus to manage and maintain its 88 breastfeeding rooms. These champions are employees who work in the departments where the rooms are located. They volunteer to promote this service and monitor the utilization of the rooms, communicating with mothers and making sure the room is kept in order (Figure 6.6).

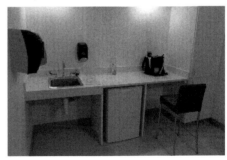

Figure 6.6 MSU Room

Additionally, the University has exceeded the requirements for nursing mothers, providing high quality, private spaces to pump breastmilk that are equipped to accommodate women's needs. MSU also provides mothers with the workplace flexibility to achieve their breastfeeding goals.

Engaging the community in ways that support nursing mothers makes MSU a leader in lactation support. The combination of education and leadership from grassroots efforts resulted in the development of accessible accommodations across campus. Lactation consultants, educators, and community providers support MSU mothers.

Michigan State University also has a long history of supporting students and employees with "family friendly" services. Examples of initiatives sponsored by the Family Resource Center include free Emergency Back-Up Child spaces, subsidized Sick Childcare in the family home, free subscription to the services of Care.Com, and student parent support with childcare scholarships, grants, peer support, and family activities. MSU also has two licensed and accredited childcare centers on campus. Breastfeeding support rounds out the array of "Lifespan" dependent care programs available to MSU students, staff, and faculty, from pregnancy to eldercare. The MSU *Work/Life Guide for Staff and Faculty* illustrates the variety of support available.

Conclusion

Michigan State University has discussed and implemented breastfeeding support strategies for forty years. Yet, as a "work in progress," there is still more that can be done. Between 2006 and 2011, the MSU Committee on Flexibility in Faculty Work/Life generated recommendations that addressed issues and concerns of faculty work and life. One of the long-term recommendations was to provide enhanced support of breastfeeding mothers by the establishment of permanent breastfeeding rooms in campus buildings.

Within a year of the passage of the federal ACA, the MSU Administration created an exemplary inventory of 88 breastfeeding rooms in 61 buildings on campus. A search tool for mothers was created as a web-based Google map to help them find rooms in various buildings across campus, and in off-campus buildings across the state of Michigan. Michigan State University strives to be a leader and has a construction standard for "Personal Health Rooms" for new and renovated buildings. This is the formal MSU policy that ensures the long-term, future support of breastfeeding mothers with the provision of rooms where they can pump/feed in private.

For some institutions it takes a federal law to "do the right thing," not unlike the Americans with Disabilities Act (ADA), Family Medical

Leave Act, and Affirmative Action laws. In 2010, the Affordable Care Act (ACA) included the provision for employers to provide workplace accommodations that enable employees who are breastfeeding to express their milk. Under Title IX, parenting or pregnant students, who may also be breastfeeding mothers on college campuses, are protected by the law, but it is up to the institutions to designate the rooms and provide the safety net and culture of support.

As the Surgeon General's Call to Action indicates, employed women have been less likely to initiate breastfeeding and tend to breastfeed for a shorter length of time than women who are not employed. Most employed mothers who are lactating have to pump milk at work for their children and need to be provided with accommodations to do so. Universities can be the workplace leaders in their communities with formal support of these mothers.

A formal policy to support breastfeeding mothers after maternity leave is an inclusive, cost-effective approach to recruit and retain the best and brightest faculty, staff, and students. It also complies with the 2010 federal healthcare law (ACA) that mandates employers with more than 50 employees to support breastfeeding mothers with appropriate space and work flexibility. Advocacy on behalf of breastfeeding students, staff, and faculty will continue at MSU. There is a plan to conduct a follow-up survey of mothers who are using the rooms and a survey of room contacts to assess the utilization and satisfaction with the program. The ongoing goal is to assess the current program satisfaction, and although it is "a work in progress," the anticipated positive feedback will reinforce MSU's commitment to a family-friendly work environment.

References

American Academy of Pediatrics (APA). (2005). *Policy Statement: Breastfeeding and the use of human milk. Pediatrics, 115* (2), 496-506. doi:10.1542/ peds.2004-2491.

Chow, T., Smithey Fulmer, I., & Olson, B. H. (2011). Perspectives of managers toward workplace breastfeeding support in the state of Michigan. *Journal of Human Lactation, 27*(2), 138-146. doi: 10.1177/0890334410391908

Chapter Seven
It Takes a Village to Feed a Child: The Johns Hopkins Breastfeeding Support Program

Michelle Carlstrom, Ian Reynolds, and Meg Stoltzfus

"First Steps" for Breastfeeding Support at Johns Hopkins

Johns Hopkins University, established in 1876 in Baltimore, Maryland, as both a teaching and research university, has long recognized the challenge for faculty and staff to achieve a healthy mix between work, personal life, and academic pursuits. While worklife programs have been part of Human Resources for many years, establishing a dedicated office in 2008—the Office of Work, Life and Engagement (referred to in this chapter as WorkLife)—bolstered attention of critical programs and policies that promote each person's work-life effectiveness. Our programs serve the faculty and staff of both Johns Hopkins University and Johns Hopkins Hospital/Health System, totaling more than 50,000 full- and part-time individuals. Among such programs is the Johns Hopkins Breastfeeding Support Program.

The Breastfeeding Support Program was formally established in 2011 in response to the Patient Protection and Affordable Care Act of 2010, but that was not the beginning of support for expressing milk in the workplace at Johns Hopkins. For years mothers had been finding creative solutions and partnerships with various departments across the institution to sustain their milk expression. From that grew a number of informal relationships, all decentralized and eventually named Lactation Services.

WorkLife's role was primarily to provide information and referrals until the first "Employee Pumping Room" opened in the Johns Hopkins Hospital. This room was and still is located in a public section of the hospital, not housed within a specialized department; however, it was staffed and owned by the Pediatrics Department, who leveraged lactation resources they used for patients to stock the employee room. WorkLife partnered with Pediatrics to provide pumps and supplies for the room that were funded by the employee benefits plan. Although the system for tracking use was rudimentary, we knew that this space was visited frequently. This began an institutional commitment to support mothers who continue breastfeeding after returning to work.

The Affordable Care Act was an opportunity for Johns Hopkins to augment its commitment to working mothers. Being able to communicate space needs as a compliance issue was the impetus for leadership discussions that ultimately rendered greater support and resources to the program. WorkLife took the message to the highest levels, from deans and financial leaders to the President of the Johns Hopkins Hospital and Health System. This attention and commitment literally opened doors to finding space in an organization where space is at a premium.

The most compelling message was not simply one of compliance, but rather a blended message that included the benefits of breastfeeding to the employer. As a healthcare and higher education environment, Johns Hopkins has long understood the benefits of breastfeeding to mother and baby, but the benefits to the employer were not fully considered until WorkLife started that conversation. Such benefits, cited for leadership, include reduced turnover, enhanced employee loyalty, lower absenteeism due to sick children, and an overall positive image of workplace support. Another key part of the message was the proposal of a shared responsibility model that would be the vehicle for opening many more Mother's Rooms across the institution. The details of this model are discussed below, but it was leadership's early approval of this model that proved to be one of the most critical factors to the program's success.

With such endorsement, it was becoming clear that Johns Hopkins needed a centrally coordinated effort for breastfeeding support and that WorkLife would lead the way, positioning the program as an employee benefit. The Johns Hopkins Breastfeeding Support Program officially launched in October 2011. A significant change from this point forward was that WorkLife would now centrally oversee all Mother's Rooms for Johns Hopkins University, Johns Hopkins Hospital, and Johns Hopkins Health System. Combining efforts in a centralized way meant managing many partnerships that ultimately led to standardized protocols of service, financial savings, and standardized reporting, while at the same time being able to support many more mothers. From the very beginning, WorkLife envisioned a holistic approach, seeking support from various stakeholders throughout the institution to develop a comprehensive Breastfeeding Support Program. We quickly fanned out to support policy development, garner financial support, plan for ample resources, educate supervisors, launch a communication campaign to reach new mothers, and take on the ever-so-important effort to identify space for new rooms. Having dedicated WorkLife professionals positioned across the institution to socialize the need, educate people on the policy, and identify solutions resulted in what is now a vibrant and growing program that serves more than 100 mothers each year, who in 2012 visited our Mother's Rooms nearly 18,000 times!

> BEST PRACTICE: The shift in oversight of lactation spaces at the University, Hospital, and Health System to be centrally located within WorkLife enabled an integrated approach culminating in a comprehensive support program for new mothers, rather than just a workplace accommodation.

The remainder of this chapter highlights the elements of our program most critical to our success: the establishment of a shared responsibility model, a strategic plan including comprehensive communication efforts, the identification and installation of Mother's Rooms across the institution, and the implementation of an accurate and inclusive data collection system.

It Takes a Village to Breastfeed a Child

Given the sheer size of Johns Hopkins, the number of employees we represent (more than 50,000 full- and part-time), and the geographic distribution of our campuses, we determined early in the process that WorkLife would not be able to manage all aspects of the Breastfeeding Support Program on our own, particularly the operation of numerous Mother's Rooms. A shared responsibility model was critical. This model takes into consideration that contributions from stakeholders across the institution are vital to achieving our desired outcomes and to the overall success of the program. Such contributions include administrative support, funding, and allocation of space for Mother's Rooms.

In the early phase of WorkLife's oversight of the Breastfeeding Support Program, a presentation outlining the rationale for and components of the program was developed and shared with leadership. These conversations provided a foundation upon which to build support for the shared responsibility model. The next step was to actually implement the model. This has been a highly rewarding and effective process, although some challenges, which will be discussed, have been encountered along the way.

> BEST PRACTICE: JHU's shared responsibility model is a unique approach to establishing day-to-day accountability for their Mother's Rooms, and to distribute some of the work involved in providing a strong university lactation support program.

The aspect of our program where the shared model is most notable is in the management of our Mother's Rooms.

Shared Funding for Mother's Rooms

Some spaces are naturally tailored to becoming a Mother's Room: they may already have a water source, convenient electrical setup, or card reader access. Spaces such as these require less time, work, and money—a fresh coat of paint and installation of privacy dividers may be all that's necessary. Other spaces demand more extensive renovation—installation of card readers, new flooring, removal of materials, and, in some instances, even demolition of walls. In either case, some funding is always necessary, and ultimately the question of "who has to pay for it?" gets raised.

While we have met with occasional resistance when requesting funding assistance, we have generally been able to identify funding sources for the creation of Mother's Rooms. The support WorkLife received from leadership at the outset has been instrumental to progress. As discussed in the opening section, meetings were scheduled early on with financial administrators and other leaders from across the institution who committed financial support to the initiative. Drawing on support at the leadership level in a strategic and thoughtful way, along with reminders that identifying space for mothers to express milk is a compliance issue, has been highly effective. Finally, we highlight the financial commitment WorkLife made to the program at the outset: to provide hospital-grade pumps in all Mother's Rooms meeting program standards (outlined later), along with the support of three WorkLife professionals tasked with ensuring the program's operation (Senior Director of Work, Life and Engagement, Director of WorkLife and Community Programs, and Breastfeeding Support Program Coordinator).

Shared Operation of Mother's Rooms

Beyond shared funding, we needed to establish a shared model for operating and maintaining the Mother's Rooms. While WorkLife remains available for general programmatic support, and mothers themselves have certain responsibilities for the space, our ultimate goal has been to identify a "room owner" for all Mother's Rooms in the program. Room owners tend to be departments located within the building in which a Mother's Room is located. The department chair or administrator typically appoints a specific individual on his or her staff to serve as point person for the program. Once a room is functional, this person assumes responsibility for the day-to-day operation of the space (checking supplies, granting access to users, etc.).

The *Mother's Room Agreement* explains in greater detail the responsibilities associated with owning a room. These responsibilities include the following:

- Ensure there is a functioning lock on the Mother's Room door;
- Arrange for registered users to receive an access code or key for the door;
- Give WorkLife staff access to the Mother's Room;
- Provide furnishings (e.g., chair, table, and wall decorations);
- Ensure that the Mother's Room is cleaned regularly, including regular trash removal;
- Purchase and stock supplies (e.g., disinfecting wipes and hand sanitizer);
- Display promotional materials provided by the Office of Work, Life and Engagement.

To emphasize the spirit of shared responsibility, the agreement also includes the obligations that WorkLife and mothers who use the space have in maintaining a Mother's Room (see Appendix for guidelines on establishing a Mother's Room, along with the complete agreement).

In addition to basic information like a program overview and the Johns Hopkins policies around expressing breastmilk in the workplace, the remainder of the guide outlines why Mother's Rooms are critical and what features they must have in order to be compliant with both the Breastfeeding Support Program and the Affordable Care Act. We share this guide during presentations and in meetings with stakeholders, and we also have it posted on our program website. It is a useful tool in steering conversations and answering questions about room ownership. As with funding, referencing the backing of leaders and compliance with the law is also helpful in conversations around room ownership. We strive to identify an owner for each new Mother's Room before it opens. In cases where this has not been possible, WorkLife "owns" the space until a permanent owner is found.

Challenges of the Shared Responsibility Model

Despite our success, there have been challenges associated with establishing a shared responsibility model. Yes, we have the support of leadership, and yes, we have the Affordable Care Act to underscore that providing space for mothers is a compliance issue. Nonetheless, a lot of persistence and perseverance is required to maintain momentum due to funding and space considerations, as well as because this initiative is outside the scope of many departments' "typical" business. Not surprisingly, some departments are less willing than others to relinquish a room in an institution where space is at a premium, not to mention the funds necessary to renovate a space.

We also knew our "identifiers" of potential space would not necessarily have the authority to release it to WorkLife. This is where it became very important to cautiously and appropriately leverage leadership support of a formally recognized program. Johns Hopkins is a large, decentralized institution, with a wide range of workplace structures and cultures. Navigating thoughtfully and sensitively can be difficult, particularly when there is pressure to open a room in an area of campus. However, these challenges can and have been overcome by communicating frequently and persuasively, identifying program "champions" around the institution, carefully drawing on leadership support as necessary, and thinking creatively.

Other Aspects of the Shared Responsibility Model

Overseeing the operation of a Mother's Room is not the only way we collectively share responsibility for the Breastfeeding Support Program. Colleagues from our fellow Human Resources offices in both the university and hospital/health system contributed to the program in part by developing policies regarding reasonable break time for nursing mothers. These policies have been immensely helpful to both mothers and supervisors. Johns Hopkins lactation specialists have also been integral to our success. While there are WorkLife professionals fully dedicated to the operation of the program, none of us are lactation experts. We are fortunate to have the support of specialists who provide a 'Warm Line' to mothers (in contrast to a "hotline," a "warm line" is a non-crisis phone number that employees can call with breastfeeding-related questions), facilitate weekly groups open to employees, offer advice regarding content for our program website, and deliver a presentation at the Johns Hopkins Baby Shower, held twice per year for expectant parents and their spouses/partners.

> BEST PRACTICE: Twice per year, WorkLife holds the Johns Hopkins Baby Shower for expectant parents and their spouses/partners to educate them about their employee benefits package and WorkLife programs and services, including the Breastfeeding Support Program.

Finally, colleagues with an interest in breastfeeding from a research perspective have been open to meeting with us to discuss potential collaboration. This is discussed in more detail later.

Mommy, Are We There Yet?

When WorkLife officially assumed responsibility for employee lactation support, we established "Breastfeeding Support Program" as the title for the program, as we felt it captured the spirit of our services. In addition to building support for the shared responsibility model, one of our first tasks was to assess where we were and outline the direction we envisioned for the program. What did we want the program to achieve and how would we get there? The following summarizes the goals we focused on when the program was first launched.

Goal One: *Support Johns Hopkins employees who choose to continue breastfeeding after returning to work following the birth of a child.* This is the premise on which the program is based. As indicated earlier, Johns Hopkins has long recognized the benefits of breastfeeding for both mothers and babies. At its core, the Breastfeeding Support Program strives to assist mothers who make this choice for themselves and their babies for as long as it is the best choice for them.

Goal Two: *Comply with the 2010 Affordable Care Act.* We took a number of steps to ensure that, as an employer, Johns Hopkins was providing reasonable break time and a place, other than a restroom, that is private and clean for mothers to express milk. We made information about the law available on our website and in other written materials about the program. We worked with Human Resources at both Johns Hopkins University and Johns Hopkins Hospital to develop and publicize policies regarding reasonable break time for nursing mothers (see Appendix for policies). Finally, as indicated previously, we recognized that success was integrally tied to opening spaces in which mothers could express milk. We worked diligently and continue to strive to establish Mother's Rooms in key areas across the institution. This is an ongoing process that will be discussed later in greater detail.

Goal Three: *Develop a master communications plan to educate expectant and new mothers, as well as the Johns Hopkins community at large, about the Breastfeeding Support Program.* In order for the program to be successful, employees must know what resources are available to them. Fortunately, at the time of the launch, our office was already known to be a source of support around many work-life issues related to family support (e.g., childcare referrals). Therefore, many employees turned to us naturally for support around breastfeeding at work. As noted earlier, we also had a very strong relationship developed with the Pediatrics Department and had already been assisting employees in certain areas of campus. Therefore, we were not starting from scratch; many working mothers already viewed us as a resource and reached out to us for one-on-one support. However, we needed to cast a wider net that would reach our multiple campuses and think more broadly about educating the entire Johns Hopkins community about the Breastfeeding Support Program. As a result, we initiated a comprehensive communications plan (described later).

Goal Four: *Educate mothers who are breastfeeding about other WorkLife services and benefits.* Working with mothers through the Breastfeeding Support Program affords us the opportunity to make them aware of other WorkLife programs and services available to them. We recognize that the needs of employees change as they age across the lifespan. Informing mothers of resources, such as childcare referrals, backup care, and parenting workshops will ideally keep them connected to our office and enable us to continue supporting them as their children grow and develop.

Goal Five: *Track use of Mother's Rooms.* Our fifth and final goal for the program was to establish a system that ensured accurate and comprehensive tracking of usage for all Mother's Rooms, the frequency of visits, and the duration of use over time. Our rationale was threefold:

1. Hard data would continue to demonstrate to leadership and stakeholders the critical need for a robust Breastfeeding Support Program;

2. The nature of the data we planned to collect would lend itself very well to research projects related to breastfeeding support in the workplace;

3. Analysis of the data would assist in evaluating the success of the program and in identifying areas of campus where the establishment of additional Mother's Rooms is necessary.

These motives will be discussed in greater detail later in the chapter, along with the actual system implemented for collecting data.

Getting the Word Out about Getting the Milk Out

One of our initial goals was to develop and launch a broad communications plan about the program. The plan included the following components:

Development of a Breastfeeding Support Program website: The site includes information about Johns Hopkins' commitment to mothers needing to express breastmilk at work; the benefits of breastfeeding to mother, child, and employer; compliance with the Affordable Care Act; guidelines for mothers, colleagues, and managers to ensure a positive outcome for all involved and affected by a mother's choice to continue breastfeeding; a list of Mother's Rooms; program components; and breastfeeding in the news.

Information for leadership and other key stakeholders: A presentation was developed and meetings scheduled with WorkLife directors and leadership across the institution. The presentation provided a rationale for the Breastfeeding Support Program and proposed the shared responsibility model under which the program would operate. As a way of generating momentum and garnering support, the presentation also highlighted positive impacts for employers resulting from breastfeeding programs. These include improved productivity and loyalty and decreased absenteeism, healthcare costs, and turnover.

Education of Supervisors. We recognize that even if mothers have a clean and secure place to express milk at work, they need to be able to have time in the midst of a busy workday to do so. To help managers understand how they can assist mothers who are breastfeeding, we have implemented several educational efforts, such as a section of our website dedicated to helping managers learn about their rights and responsibilities vis-à-vis the human resources policies at Johns Hopkins, the Federal law, and breastfeeding best practices. We also offer our services to Human Resources professionals and managers who have questions or concerns regarding employees who are breastfeeding, and we are called upon to consult on many such cases. Finally, we replicated our website content for managers into a paper reference guide, which we feel is particularly important because in many departments, such as housekeeping and nutrition, managers do not regularly have access to computers.

> BEST PRACTICE: JHU developed a Breastfeeding Support Program reference guide for managers in both electronic and print formats.

Development of a registration system to facilitate ongoing communication with mothers. Knowing who is using the Mother's Rooms and some basic information about these mothers affords the opportunity to maintain regular communication with individuals being supported by the program. Our registration form requests contact information, baby's due date, date of return to work, which Mother's Rooms they are registering for, whether the mother has breastfeed or used a breast pump, and how they learned of the Breastfeeding Support Program (see Appendix to view the form). This information is kept confidential and only shared in aggregate form for reporting purposes.

The benefits of adding a registration component are significant. After registering for the program, the mother receives an email with details about the specific rooms she registered for, information about lactation support services for mothers (breastfeeding support group and breastfeeding 'Warm Line'), and details about the Pumps for Purchase Program (discussed later). On an ongoing basis, mothers who are registered for the program receive email updates when there are changes to the program or when we open new Mother's Rooms. We can also communicate easily with the group when we receive information on topics that may be of interest to them, such as breastmilk donation.

> BEST PRACTICE: Requiring mothers to register for the Breastfeeding Support Program provides JHU with an accessible method to provide them with targeted information, as well as to collect evaluation data.

Creation of Breastfeeding Support Program signs, business cards, and licenses. Signs with a look and feel that matched other WorkLife materials were made for both the exterior and interior of Mother's Rooms. Signs include the universal symbol for breastfeeding and the address for the Breastfeeding Support Program website. Interior signs also include a welcome message for mothers and the contact information for our Breastfeeding Support Program Coordinator (see Appendix for images). (A note about signs: signage has been more challenging than we first expected because each building has its own design standards. We have used our standard Mother's Room sign where allowed and have adapted the design to fit within each individual building's standards when required to do so.)

We also designed and printed Breastfeeding Support Program business cards. These cards outline the various program components and include the program's web address. The cards are an effective tool for educating mothers and the community. We had also been made aware of 'licenses' to breast pump and breastfeed produced by the Maryland Breastfeeding Coalition and decided to replicate these for mothers to carry at Johns Hopkins (see Appendix for images).

> BEST PRACTICE: To create a consistent look for the Breastfeeding Support Program, JHU developed signs and other collateral material to post in Mother's Rooms and distribute to employees and supervisors. They strategically chose to brand the Breastfeeding Support Program in a way that complements their other WorkLife materials. Having a consistent brand strengthens their ability to introduce other WorkLife services to mothers who utilize the Breastfeeding Support Program.

Dissemination of program information through traditional channels. We rely on several communication strategies to disseminate information about various work-life initiatives, and many of these were used to get the word out about the Breastfeeding Support Program. These include email blasts, newsletters, distribution of information at events, and working with colleagues, such as HR managers and Occupational Health professionals, to educate mothers about program benefits both before and after maternity leave.

If You Build It, They Will Pump

While the communications plan was essential in giving the program momentum, we knew success rested most heavily on opening new Mother's Rooms across multiple campuses. Needless to say, in order to do so, we first needed to identify space. Asking people to give up space is a very difficult conversation at Johns Hopkins, so we understood that putting out a broad call for help was likely to be passed over. We recognized that only grass-roots efforts were going to identify the storage rooms, closets, small meeting spaces, and minimally utilized single restrooms for potential conversion into Mother's Rooms.

Before officially launching the program, we knew of a handful of rooms that existed around our many campuses, and understood that there was high demand in other areas. We immediately began identifying contacts on each campus, typically HR representatives or building managers who could help mothers find a suitable space to express milk. For many of these locations, we planned to go back later to identify a designated space, but we wanted mothers to have a place to start in the short term if they needed assistance with finding private space.

We learned quickly where there was more demand for Mother's Rooms on campus because the mothers told us. Using a five-minute travel time as a benchmark, we identified key areas on campus where large numbers of women worked, but did not have their own office space in which to pump, such as clinical areas or buildings with cubicle workspaces. We did a lot of listening to mothers, and we also began to ask users of the Mother's Rooms to attempt to identify appropriate space in the buildings where they worked.

> BEST PRACTICE: JHU uses a five-minute travel time as a benchmark to determine if there is a Mother's Room accessible to every work location.

We also reached out to staff and faculty whom we knew were supportive of WorkLife initiatives to ask them for ideas. We think of these individuals as "champions" who can contribute enormously to progress. Through interaction and stories, we learned that these champions included mothers of older, previously breastfed children, fathers of breastfed children, and individuals simply committed to meeting the work-life needs of their employees. Word began to spread as these advocates spoke with their colleagues about finding space. In many instances, we found that it was critical to find a supportive person in the facilities department. Not only do these individuals know where the empty or underutilized spaces are across campus, we discovered that they enjoy working on projects that are a little out of the ordinary.

BEST PRACTICE: Champions at JHU are mothers of older, previously breastfed children, fathers of breastfed children, and individuals simply committed to meeting the work-life needs of their employees.

Despite the fact that Johns Hopkins is a decentralized institution, we garnered leadership support to establish a cohesive program where each Mother's Room met specific criteria. Rooms that met these criteria would be eligible to receive a hospital-grade breast pump for the space, provided by WorkLife.

In keeping with Johns Hopkins' commitment to working mothers, the criteria go beyond that of the 2010 Affordable Care Act to include the following:

- Water source in the room or nearby the room;

- Dedicated solely for the purpose of expressing milk and signage outside of the room must indicate this purpose;

- Installation of an ID card reader or ID card access to allow for tracking usage (more on this later);

- Access to supplies and storage.

Although not an official requirement, we strongly prefer space that will accommodate at least two mothers at one time. Our multi-user rooms have a single entry point, but are separated into individual pumping stations by privacy curtains or some other type of divider. In our busiest rooms, WorkLife provides a hospital-grade pump in each station. In rooms with less traffic, pumps are affixed to trolleys that can move

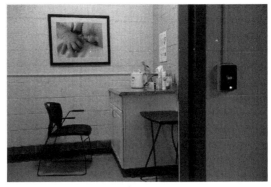

Figure 7.1 JHU Multi-User Lactation Room

between stations. This is helpful because some room users choose to bring their personal pumps, and a station without a hospital-grade pump still meets their need for a space in which to pump. Our largest room can accommodate up to five mothers at one time, but most of our rooms have two to three pumping stations (Figure 7.1).

> BEST PRACTICE: JHU provides multi-user rooms as an option to overcome scheduling challenges presented by their single-user rooms.

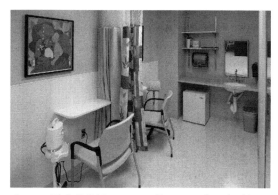

Figure 7.2 JHU Lactation Room – Single User

Single-user rooms tend to create a lot of challenges around scheduling, especially because mothers who work the same hours typically need to express milk at approximately the same time. While we are certainly open to the idea of single-user rooms and have a few of these spaces in our program, experience is teaching us to exhaust all possibilities for a multi-user room before proceeding with renovations to a space that will accommodate only one mother at a time (Figure 7.2).

Mothers, Visits, and Data, Oh My

Prior to WorkLife's oversight of the Breastfeeding Support Program, loose methods were in place for recording employee use of the employee lactation room at Johns Hopkins Hospital. A sign-in sheet attached to a clipboard was left inside the room. While mothers were expected to sign in and we believe most adhered to the process, the sign-in sheets were not used for anything beyond calculating the number of visits to the room per month to determine WorkLife's reimbursement to Pediatrics for supplies and support. Data collection was by no means a consistent practice across the institution. Before the launch of the program, mothers across Johns Hopkins were identifying their own spaces in which to express milk. There was no centralized system in place for tracking visits.

While keeping the confidentiality of users in mind, we recognized early on that capturing information around utilization and reporting it in aggregate would be extremely advantageous for three reasons:

1. Access to concrete data would enable us to underscore the importance of the initiative and the need to establish additional Mother's Rooms. We knew from our previous collaboration with the Pediatrics Department and from numerous inquiries from mothers around the institution that demand was very high. Sharing actual numbers with leadership demonstrates demand and sustains momentum for the Breastfeeding Support Program. In a given month, we track an average of 1,500 visits to our 13 fully functional Mother's Rooms (see Appendix for sample tracking spreadsheet). These numbers speak for themselves in making the case for establishing a program to meet the needs of mothers at Johns Hopkins and to be in compliance with the Affordable Care Act.

2. We realized the potential to support important research that might be conducted with our data. The information we are collecting enables us to track the number of mothers using a particular room, the number of visits a mother makes to a room per month, and how long a mother continues to express milk at work following the birth of a child. We have already identified and contacted colleagues at Johns Hopkins for whom breastfeeding support is also a priority to discuss potential research collaborations. We envision our data being valuable to research around factors that contribute to a mother's choice to breastfeed and for how long. As attention to breastfeeding support in the workplace continues to expand, our numbers might also be helpful to other organizations seeking to implement their own programs.

3. Having utilization data to analyze would be beneficial from a program evaluation standpoint as well. We hear frequently from mothers who do not have a Mother's Room in their immediate vicinity. The data we collect assists us in evaluating feedback from mothers and identifying areas of campus where demand for Mother's Rooms is especially high. Our campuses, particularly our medical campus in East Baltimore, cover a wide geographic area. This creates a significant challenge for mothers who must travel to another building to use a Mother's Room. Despite feedback from mothers, it is not always readily apparent where we will have a concentration of mothers who need breastfeeding support. Of course, this also changes over time. However, our data, along with information collected during the registration process, enables us to consider carefully where our mothers work, alongside which rooms they are

using. In turn, this highlights areas of campus to target for future Mother's Rooms. After an area of campus is identified, we can begin the process of searching for space and potential partners.

> BEST PRACTICE: Providing formal evaluation of the Breastfeeding Support Program through the collection of aggregate data, such as usage information obtained through their ID badge access to their Mother's Rooms, allows Johns Hopkins to advocate for additional spaces as needed.

Spare Parts Sold Here!

With our program now off the ground, we have been able to give attention to new components that enhance the overall quality of our program. A few of these are discussed below.

Pumps for Purchase

The Pumps for Purchase program was a relatively easy, but important addition to the Breastfeeding Support Program. It fit seamlessly into WorkLife's pre-existing Discount Programs and provided another tangible benefit to employees, particularly those who will not be using a hospital-grade pump in one of the Mother's Rooms. The breast pump manufacturers with whom we work provided us with solid guidance about how best to implement this program, including which pumps to sell, pricing, and warranty information.

As a part of this program, employees may purchase a personal breast pump at a significant discount over retail pricing. Employees may purchase discounted pumps for themselves, a spouse or partner, other family member, or a friend. WorkLife also sells accessory kits for the hospital-grade breast pumps in the Mother's Rooms at a discounted rate. To be consistent with other WorkLife discount programs, employees who earn less than $40,000 annually are eligible to receive a free accessory kit, which is compatible with a hospital-grade pump.

> BEST PRACTICE: As part of WorkLife's Discount Programs, breast pumps are sold at significantly reduced prices to Johns Hopkins faculty, staff, and students. Breast pump accessory kits that are compatible with the hospital-grade breast pumps in their Mother's Rooms are provided free to employees who earn less than $40,000 annually.

Although we have chosen to purchase rather than rent hospital-grade breast pumps to mothers for personal use, we are frequently asked about this service, and it may be something that institutions should consider when developing a breastfeeding support program.

Privacy Door Hanger

As a promotional item for the Breastfeeding Support Program, we designed a door hanger for mothers who have a private office in which to express milk. This door hanger lists information about the program, along with links to our website and the federal law (see Appendix).

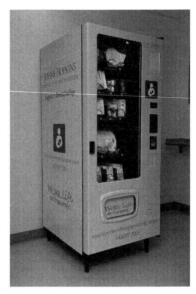

Figure 7.3 Pump Parts Vending Machine

Vending Machine for Pump Accessories

On a regular basis, we receive calls from mothers who have forgotten a piece of their accessory kit or their bottles and cannot return home to retrieve the missing piece. In our most highly utilized Mother's Rooms, we decided to provide "emergency kits" and accessory kit pieces that mothers may take on an honor system. Although this has worked fairly well, it is

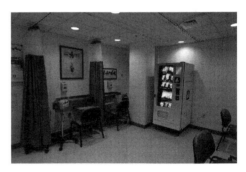

Figure 7.4 Vending Machine in Lactation Room

an added expense, and it can be a chore to ensure that emergency supplies remain stocked. We investigated retail outlets on our hospital campus that may be able to sell accessory kits or parts to mothers. However, given that the hospital is operational 24/7, this would not resolve the problem for mothers whose shifts do not coincide with the retail outlet's hours. Thus, we began researching vending machine companies that could build a custom vending machine for breast pumping supplies. We placed the machine in our highest volume Mother's Room, located at Johns Hopkins Hospital (Figures 7.3, 7.4).

138

This solution allows us to provide even more supplies to mothers at a discounted price (and at a more convenient location than WorkLife's off-site location), while also conserving the resources we spent providing emergency kits to mothers.

BEST PRACTICE: A custom vending machine for breast pump supplies was placed in our highest volume Mother's Room, located at Johns Hopkins Hospital.

"Expressing" Thanks

We are extremely grateful to Johns Hopkins for supporting WorkLife initiatives and for endorsing the Breastfeeding Support Program as a priority. This has enabled us to accomplish a great deal in the two short years WorkLife has managed the program. We are incredibly proud of the strides we have made and the support we have provided to mothers across our institution. One mother told us, "Pumping at work is such a hassle, but thanks to your efforts, it's a little bit easier! I may not even have stuck it out this long if it weren't for the Mother's Room and the peace of mind that it gives me knowing it's there when I need it."

Despite our progress, we recognize much work still lies ahead. Our primary objective at this point is to continue opening new Mother's Rooms in high-need areas. However, we also look forward to getting more involved in the national conversation on breastfeeding support. We appreciate very much the opportunity to be included in this text and know that the chapters written by other institutions will generate new ideas for and improvements to our program. We hope our collective efforts elevate attention to supporting mothers in higher education who choose to breastfeed their babies.

Chapter Eight
Future Directions for Breastfeeding on College and University Campuses

Michele L. Vancour and Michele K. Griswold

Best practices among lactation support programs are found on campuses that were expecting to move beyond simple workplace accommodations for nursing mothers to pump breastmilk by creating solutions that promoted a breastfeeding-friendly approach to lactation support. We know this is important because:

- Breastfeeding is a public health issue.

- National goals for breastfeeding persistently portray a work in progress.

- The Surgeon General issued a *Call to Action to Support Breastfeeding* and placed emphasis on workplaces supporting breastfeeding women.

- Research shows that breastfeeding is best for mothers, infants, and businesses, and to the point, workplaces need to support breastfeeding because it is the law.

- Successful, supportive breastfeeding practices exist on campuses across the country.

- Although the results are encouraging, some universities lag behind not sure where to begin, how to improve, or how to become a best practice.

Clearly, there is a shift in philosophy and culture away from unsupportive workplaces with the research that exits. Further, the shift is moving from employed mothers having to be self-advocates toward quality resources available regardless of the work setting. The foundation of this shift is rooted in the establishment of a "business case" for breastfeeding. Universities, like other workplaces, stand to realize considerable benefits from supporting their breastfeeding employees, which include lower costs, increases in productivity, and an overall greater satisfaction with employers.

Good, Better, BEST

Clearly, it is a best practice to examine best practices in place in any area in which improvement is sought, which makes this collection a much needed reference in providing lactation support in higher education. All of the universities represented in this text are excellent examples of initiative, progress, collaboration, innovation, and results. In their unique ways, each university demonstrates that institutions of higher education have the intellectual capital to make a significant change for the betterment of current and future employees (faculty and staff) and students, while simultaneously opening doors for women to achieve equality. Universities are rising above constraints to provide exemplary opportunities for their employees, including mothers, to be successful. It is possible that more universities will join the ranks of those included in the previous pages with the right amount of patience, practice, and perseverance, and lessons learned from this text. Despite the inherent differences in number of employees and students, buildings and programs, departments and acres, universities have what it takes to make lactation support programs work.

An examination of trends in lactation accommodations refers to three levels of lactation care on a continuum—awareness, support, and program (Bar-Yam, 2004). Each university represented herein demonstrated that it had progressed through the continuum to offering full-fledged lactation programs, which exceeded most popular expectations with innovative, cutting-edge offerings, like vending machines filled with breast pump supplies. However, most universities around the country find they are somewhere on the lower two-thirds of the continuum, trying to establish lactation awareness and/or striving to provide adequate lactation support.

Awareness

Beginning with the first level of the continuum, lactation awareness frequently occurs when expectant and new mothers ask employers for accommodations (Bar Yam, 2004). The federal and state laws are used as the impetus supporting their inquiries. Since there likely is no formal lactation policy and/or plan in place to direct efforts at this level, reactive accommodations often are granted on a case-by-case, informal basis. A vacant room or temporarily unoccupied space may be sanctioned for use. The breastfeeding employee uses the space to pump her milk, and figures things out, overcoming small challenges as they present. In this scenario, the mother is establishing a process to be expanded for other mothers in need in the future. New experiences like this will often help to facilitate movement from awareness to support.

Support

At the next level, lactation support, there usually is a workplace policy in place protecting a woman's right to breastfeed and receive specified accommodations, such as a private space and time to pump (Bar Yam, 2004). Within lactation support, space may be multi-use, meaning it functions as something else when not in use for lactation, or designated, meaning strictly used for lactation purposes. The time to breastfeed or pump may be established formally in a policy. There is variation across campuses with regard to the way this time is used. Some universities offer women paid time to breastfeed or pump, while other universities consider this time as unpaid, comp time, or personal leave time. Once universities have strong lactation supports in place, they are more than halfway to establishing a lactation program.

Lactation Program

The last level on the continuum is an institutionalized lactation program. This level includes all of those important elements of lactation awareness and support, and adds to them the details that make a lactation program run efficiently and effectively. Any space designated for lactation purposes is fully equipped with the essentials (comfortable chair, privacy, a sink, an electrical outlet, access to a lactation consultant, flexible time/schedule to pump as needed). Additionally, lactation programs provide a well-stated policy, access to a breast pump (either provided, for sale, or for rent) and/or supplies, and education. Many of these universities also have onsite or nearby childcare centers and encourage women to breastfeed their babies as needed during the day (Bar-Yam, 2004).

Space, Time, Education, and Support

A comprehensive lactation program is framed around four essential components: space, time, education, and support (U.S. Department of Health and Human Services [USDHHS], n.d.; Carothers & Hare, 2010). Even on campuses with the greatest number of designated lactation spaces, space is still an issue. Recently, the University of Michigan, for example, invested in a plan to improve and expand its lactation spaces, ultimately increasing its spaces from 60 to 83 across their campus (J. McAlpine, personal communication, July 31, 2013). It is a best practice to have a plan for renovation of existing buildings and the creation of new buildings that includes consideration of lactation spaces to maintain the five-minute walking rule. This rule also takes into consideration the constraints placed on some women who cannot use their offices, may not have private offices, and/or may feel vulnerable or lack adequate privacy where they work.

Space is intricately related to time, which primarily refers to the time spent pumping breastmilk. However, the time component also includes the time spent traveling to and from the designated space. Therefore, it makes good business sense that designated lactation spaces be located within a reasonable amount of time or walking distance from the mothers who will use them. As such, many universities have established a five-minute walking rule. This is quickly becoming a commonly adopted rule, since campuses often are spread out and occupy more than one building. The University of California Davis uses a calculated route (calculated at two miles per hour or about 800 feet) to help identify spaces and provide convenient access to nursing mothers on their campus.

From the employer perspective, the time an employee spends away from her "work" may be the focal point, but for many mothers, finding the time to pump within a full scheduled day may prove to be a greater challenge than imagined. It is important that all angles be considered in planning lactation programs to increase positive outcomes. The nature of academia involves meetings, classes, and full schedules of activities regardless of the role (employee/student) and position, and some women find it hard to get away to pump, which is a barrier to breastfeeding and meeting personal and national goals. However, this struggle is lessened on campuses that have a supportive culture.

Supportive culture and education can go hand-in-hand. Johns Hopkins found an innovative method to deliver important pre- and postnatal education through its popular Baby Shower. New and expectant parents who attend the Baby Shower learn about breastfeeding support, childcare, their employee health benefits package, and other relevant topics.

Over the past twenty years, universities have become more family-friendly through their work-life offerings and attempts to maintain a competitive advantage in recruiting and retaining their employees, which is favorable to lactation services. However, one of the biggest hurdles to transitioning through the continuum is a campus culture that supports breastfeeding as a family and business value. Since support can be received through different methods, it is important that a consistent message permeate the campus environment.

144

"Good, better, best. Never let it rest. Until your good is better and your better is best."

Getting to Good

The number of universities providing "good" lactation programs is encouraging. With the passage of the federal law in 2011, some universities stepped up their efforts adding lactation to their menu of family-friendly offerings. A quick "Google" search of 'university and lactation program' produced a list of over three million hits. Links to University of Rhode Island, Columbia University, University of California San Diego, University of California Berkeley, Tulane University, Washington State University, University of Virginia, University of California Davis, Cornell University, University of Michigan, and Wichita State University are among the top results. It is good news to see campuses with links to lactation programs, because website promotion of lactation programs is essential for providing basic information and resources to everything a nursing mother needs. Breastfeeding education via newsletters and other promotional materials is an excellent addition to lactation program websites, too. These items offer support and are accessible on an as-needed basis.

Better for Babies and Business

Universities with lactation programs that are better than the rest tend to offer a wider range of support, and find creative ways to integrate breastfeeding into their campus culture. An important caveat worth sharing is that there isn't always a one-size-fits-all approach when it comes to finding what works. A good example is found in the variations in room scheduling that occurs among lactation programs. Some campuses have ever only used an "access as needed" approach, and claim it works perfectly. Whereas, some campuses rely on paper sign-up sheets or informal wall calendars posted outside or inside rooms, which are managed by the women using the rooms. While others invest in more sophisticated scheduling options, like the Google calendar used by George Washington University. Other noteworthy differences are found among funding streams, management (centralized vs. decentralized) systems, and partnerships. The trick is finding what works for your program and university.

Partnerships seem to make the difference when it comes to valuable resources. Lactation programs benefit from relationships with diverse members of their campus communities, health professionals affiliated with medical schools and hospitals, and leaders from off campus. Some universities find creative ways to partner. Several campuses identify champions on their campuses to help manage lactation spaces.

145

Others work with faculty, students, and medical professionals to provide research, evaluation, and lactation consultations. Still others reach out to their state breastfeeding coalitions for resources and education on becoming breastfeeding-friendly workplaces.

Best Practices Set the Standard for the Future

Several universities' lactation programs truly are best, having exceeded the expectations involved in offering a lactation program. They are providing innovative additions, gaining attention, and reaping the rewards. These universities have reached for the stars and find themselves among the best. Five of these programs are showcased in this text, and some of their exceptional practices are noted below, along with a few others.

- The University of Michigan has invested in breastfeeding best practices and continues to strive to find new and innovative approaches. Among several best practices, their website includes a **rating system** of their lactation spaces: *"1 Star (*) = available for use but does not meet ACA guidelines and is not recommended by the Work/Life Resource Center, to 5 Stars (*****) = highly recommended by the Work/Life Resource Center" (University of Michigan, 2014).*

- *The University of Washington has more than 15 lactation stations on their campus. Their* **detailed website** *lists the following information for each space: the location, the contact including information on orientation, scheduling, key or key-code assignment, hours of operation, appliances (e.g., refrigeration, hospital-grade pumps), and a description of the accommodations (University of Washington, 2014).*

- The University of California Davis and George Washington University tied their lactation programs into their campuses' **sustainability** approaches. They are capitalizing on the fact that breastfeeding is naturally "lean, green, and clean," carrying this theme throughout their lactation programs.

- A **key partnership** between Tulane University's Mary Amelia Douglas-Whited Community Women's Health Education Center and the Louisiana Breastfeeding Coalition led to their breastfeeding program. Further support from The Tulane University Women's Center and the Louisiana WIC program resulted in additional spaces, demonstrating the importance of community collaborations (Tulane Breastfeeding Program, 2014).

- **Accessory kits** are a hot commodity on some campuses that have found ways to make these items accessible. Many universities sell kits through their health services' pharmacy or bookstore, and/or maintain links to online retailers on their websites. Most noteworthy is Johns Hopkins University's vending machine, stocked with discounted accessory kits that can be purchased 24 hours a day.

- Sharing **lessons learned** is rooted in the philosophy of higher education. The University of Rhode Island is at the forefront, documenting and publicly sharing valuable lessons they learned along the way as they planned and implemented their lactation program. They created the guide, *College and University Lactation Programs: Some Additional Considerations*, with resources to help other universities provide lactation programs.

- With **technology** offering an easily accessible format for society, a few universities are looking to expand their services through Apps. One university is trying to create an App that will identify the location of their 83 lactation spaces.

- **Awards** are a great reward. Almost all of the universities represented in this text have been recognized with awards on their outstanding lactation programs, making them model programs. These universities availed themselves of these opportunities by reaching out to their local and state breastfeeding coalitions and taking advantage of their resources.

Always Room for Improvement

One area for concentrated improvement in lactation support programs in higher education is evaluation. Aside from collecting basic room usage information, not much else is being captured with regard to women's experiences combining breastfeeding and work in this setting. Tracking usage has its benefits. It identifies the number of women using the rooms, the number of their visits, and length of time each woman spends in the room. It also identifies trends around popular times of day for pumping, which can be beneficial for making the case that additional rooms are needed. Universities tracking usage either do so via their card swipe room access or pen-and-paper.

However, there is great value in investing time and resources in more in-depth evaluations. Evaluation criteria can be designed to examine the extent to which lactation program objectives are being met, as well as to ascertain the impact of lactation support efforts on breastfeeding practices. The results can provide insight into the state of the program (how many users, how many times, how many hours), as well as priorities for resources (what needs improvement), training and education needs (supervisors' support, flexibility for breaks), and overall quality of services (available, comfortable, clean, and convenient spaces). They also can give employers information on absenteeism, turnover, and healthcare costs. Self-report surveys from mothers may provide a glimpse into universities' abilities to support breastfeeding mothers through their return to work, providing evidence to measure against Healthy People 2020 objectives. Best practices in evaluation would include a variety of methods for gaining process and outcome data to support lactation programs and breastfeeding.

Making Mothers' Milk Matter

Recent media events document the professional perils academic mothers may encounter if their educational institutions do not provide lactation and other support for women to achieve success. Academic mothers know firsthand the potential implications involved in "make-do" situations. Occurrences illustrate how little progress has taken place in higher education and society in the years since women joined the workforce. The demands of motherhood push many academic mothers against the maternal wall (Williams, 2004), preventing them from progressing through the "pipeline" (Mason & Goulden, 2002; Mason & Goulden, 2004; Vancour, 2012) in terms of their career advancement and overall progress. Research has correlated mothers' hindered career advancement to unsupportive work environments (Vancour & Sherman, 2010). Campuses, like the University of Rhode Island, recognize that efforts need to focus on strategies that support women's work, and they secured grants to provide strategic solutions for early to mid-career scientists and women in STEM. However, there is more work to be done in this area in order to prevent nuisances (pumping in unsanitary and noisy toilet stalls; leaking breastmilk while teaching because there was not time in a busy schedule or an adequate, private space to pump; pumping in cars in parking lots, or worse, pumping while driving to and from work) associated with breastfeeding that have been the experiences of too many women in academia (Vancour, 2012).

The responsibility for preventing similar future occurrences in academia lie with universities not mothers. National data shows that mothers are initiating breastfeeding at birth at higher rates than ever, but workplace environments are not conducive to maintaining a breastfeeding lifestyle when they return to work. Lactation programs are essential to a strong work-life agenda. It is time to develop new ideas and make improvements to lactation programs to improve support for mothers in higher education that choose to breastfeed their babies.

References

Bar-Yam, N. B. (2004). Corporate and maternal strategies to support lactation in the workplace. *Journal of the Association for Research on Mothering, 6*(2), 127-138.

Carothers, C., & Hare, I. (2010). The business case for breastfeeding. *Breastfeeding Medicine, 5*(5), 229-231. doi: 10.1089/bfm.2010.0046

Mason, M. A. & Goulden, M. (2002, November/December). Do babies matter? The effect of family formation on the lifelong careers of academic men and women. [Electronic version]. *Academe, 88* (6).

Mason, M. A. & Goulden, M. (2004, November/December). Do babies matter (part II)? Closing the baby gap. *Academe, 90* (2), 10-15.

Tulane University. (2014). *Tulane Breastfeeding Program*. Retrieved May 18, 2014 from http://womenshealth.tulane.edu/pages/detail/84/Tulane-Breastfeeding-Program.

U. S. Department of Health and Human Services (USDHHS), Health Resources Services Administration (HRSA), Maternal Child Health Bureau (n.d.) *Business case for breastfeeding*. Retrieved January 19, 2014 from http://mchb.hrsa.gov/pregnancyandbeyond/breastfeeding/

University of Michigan Work/Life Resource Center . (2014). *Parenting and lactation resources – lactation rooms at U-M Ann Arbor*. Retrieved January 19, 2014 from http://hr.umich.edu/worklife/parenting/lactationrooms.html

University of Washington. (2014). *Campus lactation stations*. Retrieved May 18, 2014 from http://depts.washington.edu/womenctr/services-resources/campus-lactation-stations/

Vancour, M.L. & Sherman, W.M. (2010, August). Academic life balance for mothers: Pipeline or pipe dream? In A. O'Reilly (Ed.), *Mothering at the 21st century: Identity, policy, experience and agency*. New York, NY: Columbia University Press.

Vancour, M. L. (2012). Academic mothers climb the ladder of promotion and tenure one rung at a time. In L. O. Hallstein & A. O'Reilly (Eds.). *Academic*

Motherhood in a Post-Second Wave Context: Challenges, Strategies and Possibilities. Bradford, Ontario: Demeter Press.

Williams, J. (2004, November/December). Hitting the maternal wall. *Academe, 90* (2), 16-20.

Appendices

Ten Steps to Successful Breastfeeding

URI Marketing Flier

URI Lactation Policy

UC Davis Chancellor Letter and Lactation Facility Standards

UC Davis Chancellor Letter and Policy on Lactation Accommodation

JH Establishing a Mothers Room

JH Mother's Room Agreement form

JH Hospital and University Policies on Break Time

JH Breastfeeding Support Program Registration form

JH Mother's Room sign

JH Breastfeeding Support flier

JH Breastfeeding Support Business Card

JH Breastfeeding License

JH Tracking Spreadsheet

JH Door Hanger

Resources

10 STEPS TO SUCCESSFUL BREASTFEEDING

1. MAINTAIN A WRITTEN BREASTFEEDING POLICY THAT IS ROUTINELY COMMUNICATED TO ALL HEALTH CARE STAFF.

2. TRAIN ALL HEALTH CARE STAFF IN SKILLS NECESSARY TO IMPLEMENT THIS POLICY.

3. INFORM ALL PREGNANT WOMEN ABOUT THE BENEFITS AND MANAGEMENT OF BREASTFEEDING.

4. HELP MOTHERS INITIATE BREASTFEEDING WITHIN ONE HOUR OF BIRTH.

5. SHOW MOTHERS HOW TO BREASTFEED AND HOW TO MAINTAIN LACTATION, EVEN IF THEY ARE SEPARATED FROM THEIR INFANTS.

6. GIVE INFANTS NO FOOD OR DRINK OTHER THAN BREAST MILK, UNLESS MEDICALLY INDICATED.

7. PRACTICE "ROOMING IN"—ALLOW MOTHERS AND INFANTS TO REMAIN TOGETHER 24 HOURS A DAY.

8. ENCOURAGE UNRESTRICTED BREASTFEEDING.

9. GIVE NO PACIFIERS OR ARTIFICIAL NIPPLES TO BREASTFEEDING INFANTS.

10. FOSTER THE ESTABLISHMENT OF BREASTFEEDING SUPPORT GROUPS AND REFER MOTHERS TO THEM ON DISCHARGE FROM THE HOSPITAL OR CLINIC.

(BABY-FRIENDLY USA, N.D.)

URI WORK-LIFE DAY
Tuesday, Oct. 27, 2009

Today, balancing work, life, and family affects **everyone.**

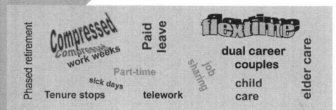

Phased retirement · Compressed work weeks · Tenure stops · Part-time · sick days · telework · Paid leave · job sharing · flextime · dual career couples · child care · elder care

October is National Work-Family Month. To acknowledge the importance of work-life balance for today's workers and students, as well as the significant strides URI has made in promoting a flexible, life- and family-friendly place to work and study for men and women, we ask you to join us during URI **Work-Life Day**. Events include a lunchtime film, a brown bag lunch discussion, and tours of the Lactation Rooms for new mothers. In particular, please join us for the main event at 3:00 p.m., during which URI will receive a Gold "*Breastfeeding Friendly Workplace Award*" from the Rhode Island Department of Health, followed by a keynote address from work-life expert, **Ann Higginbotham, Distinguished Professor of History**, Eastern Conn. State University, and Chair of the AAUP Committee of Women. Prof. Higginbotham writes and speaks extensively on the history of women, work, and family. A wine and cheese reception will follow.

9:00 - 10:00	Tours of Mother's Room - *001 Carlotti Hall - please drop by*
11:30 - 12:30	Film: *The Motherhood Manifesto* - *Memorial Union, Atrium 11*
12:30 - 1:30	Brown Bag Lunch: "*Parents Returning to Work:/School: Issues & Resources*" - *318 Memorial Union* (fruit/cookies provided)
1:30 - 2:30	Tours of Mother's Room - *001 Carlotti Hall - please drop by*
3:00 - 4:00	Award Ceremony & Keynote Address - *UClub Rhode Island Room* ~ Rhode Island 2009 Breastfeeding Friendly Workplace Award Remarks: Robert Weygand; Helen Mederer; RI Dept. of Health ~ Keynote: Ann Higginbotham, Professor of History, Eastern Connecticut State University: "*Why Family Friendly Matters*"
4:00 - 5:00	Reception - *UClub Rhode Island Room*

Sponsored by the NSF ADVANCE Program, the Elsevier Foundation, the URI Women's Center, and the URI Work-Life Committee

URI LACTATION POLICY

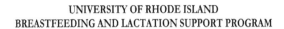

UNIVERSITY OF RHODE ISLAND
BREASTFEEDING AND LACTATION SUPPORT PROGRAM

Originators: ADVANCE Office & URI Work-Life Committee
Date: November 20, 2008
Policy #08-1

Purpose:
The University of Rhode Island recognizes the importance and benefits of breastfeeding for both mothers and their infants, and in promoting a family-friendly work and study environment. Rhode Island Law provides for the needs of mothers who are nursing and their infants, as outlined in the End Note of this policy, and URI intends to fully comply with these provisions of state law by implementing a breastfeeding and lactation policy for students, faculty, and staff.

By implementing a breastfeeding and lactation policy, the University strives to create an exceptional environment conducive to working and learning and attuned to both professional and personal needs, such as the needs of a mother who is nursing to feed and/or to express milk for her baby while she is at work or school.

Applicable To:
All female University faculty, staff, and students.

Responsibility:
All University supervisors are responsible for being aware of the policy and working with female employees to arrange mutually convenient lactation break times. The Office of Student Affairs will be responsible for making this policy known to female students.

Policy:
The University of Rhode Island recognizes the importance and benefits of breastfeeding for both mothers and their infants, and in promoting a family-friendly work and study environment. Therefore, in accordance with Rhode Island state law, the University of Rhode Island acknowledges that a woman may breastfeed her child in any place open to the public on campus, and shall provide sanitary and private space, other than a toilet stall, in close proximity to the work or study area for employees or students who are nursing to be used as a lactation room. Supervisors/chairs will work with employees who are nursing to schedule reasonable and flexible break times each day for this activity.

    1.   **Lactation Breaks**

    a)   Whenever possible, the University shall provide flexibility for staff and faculty mothers who give their Department Chair or Supervisor adequate notice identifying a need for lactation support and facilities.

    b)   Mothers are responsible for requesting lactation support prior to or during maternity leave, preferably no later than two weeks before returning to work.

    c)   The unpaid time (such as a lunch period), generally not to exceed one hour, ideally should run concurrently with an employee's paid break time (if applicable), but the University shall make separate time available, if this is not reasonable. Supervisors and employees shall work together to establish mutually convenient times.

    d)   Alternatively, personal leave, vacation time, or flexible scheduling may be used for this accommodation.

e)   It is assumed that no serious disruption of University operations will result from providing lactation time.

f)   Consistent with URI's efforts to recognize the importance of supporting the needs of working caregivers, supervisors will respond seriously, positively, and will ensure that there are no negative consequences to mothers who are nursing when lactation break times are needed.

g)   Students and instructors planning to use lactation facilities must do so around their scheduled class times.   Although any necessary student accommodations should be negotiated with individual professors, professors are not required to excuse tardiness or absences due to lactation needs.

2.   Lactation Facilities
a)   The University of Rhode Island shall provide sanitary and private facilities in close proximity to the work area across campus for mothers to breastfeed or to express breast milk.

b)   The location may be the place an employee normally works if there is adequate privacy, cleanliness, and is comfortable for the employee.

c)   Areas such as restrooms are not considered appropriate spaces for lactation purposes, unless the restroom is equipped with a separate, designated room for lactation purposes.

Procedure:

1.   Supervisors who receive a lactation accommodation request should review available space in their department/unit and be prepared to provide appropriate nearby space and break time.

2.   If the employee or student wishes to use designated lactation rooms, they are listed at http://www.uri.edu/advance/work_life_support/lactation_facilities.html. Included are descriptions of each lactation room, what, if any, pumping equipment is available, and whether provisions for the appropriate storage of breast milk are provided.

3.   Mothers who are breastfeeding or expressing milk shall be responsible for keeping the facilities clean, and, where pumps are available, for cleaning and sanitizing the breast pumps after each use.

4.   If an employee has comments, concerns, or questions regarding the URI Breastfeeding and Lactation Support Program Policy or other work-life balance personnel policies, she or he should contact the Office of Human Resources at (401)874-2416. Those who believe they have been denied appropriate accommodation or need assistance on how to make or respond to a request for accommodation should contact the Office of Human Resources at (401)874-2416. Students and others who have questions regarding access and use of the lactation facilities or would like general information about breastfeeding in the workplace and other work-life balance topics may contact the ADVANCE Office at (401) 874-9422.

UNIVERSITY OF CALIFORNIA

BERKELEY • DAVIS • IRVINE • LOS ANGELES • MERCED • RIVERSIDE • SAN DIEGO • SAN FRANCISCO   SANTA BARBARA • SANTA CRUZ

1111 Franklin Street
Oakland, California 94607-5200
Phone: (510) 987-9074
Fax:(510) 987-9086
http://www.ucop.edu

August 23, 2013

CHANCELLORS
LAWRENCE BERKELEY NATIONAL LABORATORY DIRECTOR
MEDICAL CENTER CHIEF EXECUTIVE OFFICERS

Dear Colleagues:

As part of our commitment to a workplace culture supportive of family care-giving responsibilities, and in recognition of the importance and benefits of breastfeeding for both mothers and their infants, the University established the staff policy on Accommodations for Nursing Mothers (PPSM 84) which was released last month.

This month I am sharing with you the Lactation Facility Standards for the UC Community developed by the UC Systemwide Advisory Committee on the Status of Women (SACSW) in collaboration with UCOP Systemwide Employee Relations. These Standards establish guidelines for lactation facilities across the system.

In addition, I am sponsoring an annual Lactation Accommodation Award to recognize locations that provide exceptional support to nursing mothers. An announcement of the Award program will be sent out this month, along with the Lactation Facility Standards. Information will be posted on the UC Living Well website and distributed to key stakeholders throughout the system. In early spring 2014, locations will be contacted and asked to self nominate for the first annual Lactation Facility Recognition Award.

With this award, the UC would be joining many other public, private, and governmental organizations that support nursing mothers.

With best wishes,

Sincerely yours,

Mark G. Yudof
President

LACTATION FACILITY STANDARDS FOR THE UC COMMUNITY

Criteria	Minimum Requirement — Basic	Recognition Levels — Silver	Recognition Levels — Gold
Place	Private, sanitary space (not a toilet stall). Equipped with lighting, a table, comfortable chair, and electrical outlet. Lactation spaces located in close proximity to a nursing mothers work area.	Same as Basic, plus: Private rooms that lock from the inside. A source of hot running water is within close proximity or in the room. Rooms are within a 5 minute walk from work area. Sanitary or disinfectant wipes are available for cleaning spills and hands.	Same as Silver, plus: A hospital grade electric pump may be available for use on campus. When required for certain types of jobs, where time/logistical constraints make it difficult to leave the building, a room equipped at least with basic level requirements is located within the building.
Time	A reasonable amount of time. Break times will be at mutually-agreeable times, no fewer than twice per day. The break includes the time associated with travel, expressing milk, clean-up, and storage.	Same as Basic, plus: Break times will be at mutually agreeable times up to three times per day.	Same as Silver, plus: Break times will be at mutually agreeable times up to three times per day. Process in place to request additional flexibility if required.
Access	Webpage with information to show location of lactation rooms, how to register to use and access the rooms. Lactation facilities should be easily found by search engines on the location's websites. Lactation facilities should be clearly labeled and located in accessible areas.	Same as Basic, plus: A method to indicate that room is in use, for example a sign-in sheet or dry erase board with time being used (ie., 10:00am - 10:20am).	Same as Silver, plus: Reservation mechanism, e.g. web-based system or other sign up system for reserving rooms (to ensure room availability when arrive to use it).

Establishing Lactation Facility Standards and a Recognition Program for the UC Community

UC Systemwide Advisory Committee on the Status of Women

The UC Systemwide Advisory Committee on the Status of Women (SACSW) was established in May 2008 to examine issues regarding the status of women staff, students and faculty at the University of California; to analyze existing policies, procedures, and/or programs that affect those issues; to serve as a coordinating body for campus, Office of the President and Lawrence Berkeley National Laboratory Committees on the Status of Women; to identify model programs or activities and support systemwide implementation; and to recommend to the President changes that will continue to afford women equal and fair access to campus programs, activities and opportunities.

In its 2010 inaugural report, SACSW addressed three major themes – "Work/Life," "Workforce Development," and "Data Analysis." Under "Work/Life" the committee made the following recommendations to the President regarding lactation facilities:

- Lactation rooms should be funded and adequately administered with someone in the local UC structure clearly denoted as responsible for the program.
- Lactation facilities should be clearly labeled as such and located in accessible areas.
- Lactation facilities and programs should be widely advertised and information about them should be easily found by search engines on the location's websites.
- Nursing women should have access to a comfortable, private, lockable room within a 5 minute walk from their work location. Lactation rooms should be equipped with breast pumps and refrigeration.
- All UC locations should commit to making lactation stations available in existing buildings, and during planning phases, provide for lactation stations in all new UC buildings.

In 2012, President Yudof charged SACSW with developing a strategy to publicly recognize locations that are providing exceptional support to nursing mothers.

Lactation accommodation has been an ongoing project for SACSW and we are pleased to make this recommendation to the President.

In the spirit of enhancing UC's goal to be a family-friendly work place and to support the University's ability to recruit and retain the most qualified female faculty and staff, as well as the most outstanding students, SACSW recommends that the President establish Lactation Facility Standards and sponsor an annual Lactation Accommodation Award to recognize locations that provide exceptional support to nursing mothers.

Inaugural Announcement

SACSW is recommending that President Yudof announce the Lactation Facility Standards and the Recognition Program in mid-August (2013). Information will be posted on the UC Living Well website and distributed to key stakeholders (Wellness/Health Centers, Benefits Offices, Human Resource Offices, Academic Personnel Departments, and Student Services) throughout the system.

In early spring 2014, locations will be contacted and asked to self nominate to receive the first annual Lactation Facility Recognition Program award in the spring of 2014.

Lactation Facility Standards for the UC Community and Recognition Program

The Lactation Facility Standards are comprised of four criteria: Place, Time, Access, and Education. Under California State Labor Law, each location is required to meet the minimum requirements – "to make a reasonable effort to provide employees with the use of a room or other location, other than a toilet stall, in close proximity to the employee's work area, for the employee to express milk in private."

In the attached standards, SACSW has identified additional criteria beyond the minimum requirements. Many locations have made tremendous strides in providing quality lactation facilities and information to nursing mothers. Establishing systemwide standards and a recognition program will continue to promote the University of California as a family-friendly workplace and recognize the efforts of locations to support nursing mothers.

Process for Selection

Annually in early spring, the Vice President of Human Resources will send out a call asking all locations to self-nominate based on the Lactation Facility Standards criteria posted on the SACSW and UC Living Well websites. Materials submitted by the locations will be reviewed by a subcommittee comprised of SACSW members and Systemwide Employee Relations staff.

The winning location(s) will be announced the following month and will receive a recognition letter from the President and be publicly recognized systemwide through the systemwide newsletter, *Our University*, as well as recognition on the UC Living Well site and on the local wellness site(s) at the winning location(s).

What is required to have a recognition program?

Policy Changes
- The standards of this recognition program are consistent with the newly issued policy, Accommodations for Nursing Mothers – PPSM 84. Therefore we do not anticipate any immediate policy changes to implement this recognition program.

Website Enhancement
- UCOP HR and Internal Communications will add a "lactation accommodation" section to At Your Service and the Wellness websites. The section would educate employees about their rights, link employees to resources available systemwide as well as to resources at their locations. The Lactation Facility Standards and the checklist for the recognition program will also be posted on both websites.

Measuring Success

As part of the Lactation Facility Standards, SACSW recommends that locations collect simple data to document the progress and value of the lactation support program. This data can be used by each location to measure the success of the program and for ongoing program improvement.

Locations will be encouraged to obtain feedback from women who use the facilities. Typical questions will measure satisfaction with the lactation room accommodations, the availability of the room when needed, the willingness of supervisors to provide needed flexibility for milk expression breaks, and the usefulness of resources or materials.

UC DAVIS CHANCELLOR LETTER AND POLICY ON LACTATION ACCOMMODATION

UNIVERSITY OF CALIFORNIA

BERKELEY • DAVIS • IRVINE • LOS ANGELES • MERCED • RIVERSIDE • SAN DIEGO • SAN FRANCISCO   SANTA BARBARA • SANTA CRUZ

1111 Franklin Street
Oakland, California 94607-5200
Phone: (510) 987-9074
Fax:(510) 987-9086
http://www.ucop.edu

July 3, 2013

CHANCELLORS
LAWRENCE BERKELEY NATIONAL LABORATORY DIRECTOR
MEDICAL CENTER CHIEF EXECUTIVE OFFICERS

Dear Colleagues:

Enclosed is the University of California Personnel Policy for Staff Members 84: Accommodations for Nursing Mothers.

As part of our commitment to a workplace culture supportive of family care-giving responsibilities, and in recognition of the importance and benefits of breastfeeding for both mothers and their infants, the University established the staff policy on Accommodations for Nursing Mothers.

Under the provisions of this policy, and in compliance with State and federal law, the University will provide:

- appropriate sanitary and private space for lactation purposes, in close proximity to the nursing mother's work area; and

- a reasonable amount of break time to accommodate the needs of nursing mothers.

I would like to acknowledge the commitment and support of the Systemwide Advisory Committee on the Status of Women (SACSW) for the creation of this policy.

The staff policy on Accommodations for Nursing Mothers is effective as of this date and will be published online at http://policy.ucop.edu/.

Sincerely yours,

Mark G. Yudof
President

Enclosure

cc: Members, President's Cabinet
       Chief Human Resource Officers
       University Policy Office

Accommodations for Nursing Mothers

Responsible Officer:	Vice President – Human Resources
Responsible Office:	Human Resources
Issuance Date:	
Effective Date:	
Scope:	Professional & Support Staff, Managers & Senior Professionals, and Senior Management Group members.

I.   POLICY SUMMARY

In promoting a family-friendly work environment, the University of California recognizes the importance and benefits of breastfeeding for both mothers and their infants. The University will make private space available for lactation purposes and will provide lactation break periods for employees who are breastfeeding (hereinafter referred to as "nursing mothers").

II.   DEFINITIONS

Exception to Policy: An action that exceeds what is allowable under current policy or that is not expressly provided for under policy. Any such action must be treated as an exception.

Executive Officer: The University President, Chancellor, or Laboratory Director.

Exempt Employee: An employee who, based on duties performed and manner of compensation, is exempt from the Fair Labor Standards Act (FLSA) minimum wage and overtime provisions. Because of hourly pay practices, an employee appointed to a per diem position in an exempt title will be treated as a non-exempt employee subject to FLSA minimum wage and overtime provisions.

Exempt employees shall be paid an established monthly or annual salary and are expected to fulfill the duties of their positions regardless of hours worked. Exempt employees are not eligible to receive overtime compensation or compensatory time off, and are not required to adhere to strict time, record keeping, and attendance rules for pay purposes. Exempt titles are identified in Universitywide title and pay plans.

Non-exempt Employee: An employee who, based on duties performed and manner of compensation, is subject to all FLSA provisions. Because of hourly pay practices, an employee appointed to a per diem position shall be treated as a non-exempt employee subject to FLSA minimum wage and overtime provisions.

Non-exempt employees shall be required to account for time worked on an hourly and fractional hourly basis and are to be compensated for qualified overtime hours at the premium (time-and-one-half) rate. Non-exempt titles are identified in title and pay plans.

Top Business Officer: Executive Vice President–Business Operations for the Office of the President, Vice Chancellor for Administration, or the position responsible for the location's financial reporting and payroll as designated by the Executive Officer.

III. POLICY TEXT

A.   *Lactation Facilities*
The University will provide, in close proximity to the nursing mother's work area, appropriate sanitary and private space with a table, electrical outlet, and comfortable chair.

B.   *Lactation Break Period*
The University will provide a reasonable amount of break time to accommodate the needs of nursing mothers.

  1.   Exempt employees:
       In accordance with PPSM 31 – Hours of Work, the time provided for lactation break periods does not need to be recorded.

  2.   Non-exempt employees:

       If possible the nursing mother's lactation break period should be concurrent with her rest period. If the lactation break period cannot run concurrently with the existing rest period, the University will make separate lactation break time available. The separate lactation break period will be unpaid.

Supervisors are encouraged to allow flexible scheduling, whenever possible, to accommodate lactation breaks.

No negative employment actions will be taken when requests for accommodation are made pursuant to this policy.

C. *Other Reasonable Accommodation*
The University will provide other reasonable accommodation or transfer to a less strenuous or hazardous position upon receipt of information from the nursing mother's

health care provider stating that a reasonable accommodation or transfer is medically advisable.

IV. COMPLIANCE / RESPONSIBILITIES

A. Implementation of the Policy
The Vice President–Human Resources is the Responsible Officer for this policy and has the authority to implement the policy. The Responsible Officer may apply appropriate interpretations to clarify the policy provided that the interpretations do not result in substantive changes to the underlying policy. The Chancellor is authorized to establish and is responsible for local procedures necessary to implement the policy.

B. Revisions to the Policy
The President is the Policy Approver and has the authority to approve policy revisions upon recommendation by the Vice President–Human Resources.

The Vice President–Human Resources has the authority to initiate revisions to the policy, consistent with approval authorities and applicable *Bylaws* and *Standing Orders* of the Regents.

The Executive Vice President–Business Operations has the authority to ensure that policies are regularly reviewed, updated, and consistent with other governance policies.

C. Approval of Actions
Actions within this policy must be approved in accordance with local procedures. Chancellors and the Vice President–Human Resources are authorized to determine responsibilities and authorities at secondary administrative levels in order to establish local procedures necessary to implement this policy.

All actions applicable to PPSM-covered staff employees who are not Senior Management Group members that exceed this policy, or that are not expressly provided for under any policy, must be approved by the Vice President–Human Resources.

D. Compliance with the Policy
The following roles are designated at each location to implement compliance monitoring responsibility for this policy:

The Top Business Officer and/or the Executive Officer at each location will designate the local management office to be responsible for the ongoing reporting of policy compliance.

The Executive Officer is accountable for monitoring and enforcing compliance mechanisms and ensuring that monitoring procedures and reporting capabilities are established.

The Vice President–Human Resources is accountable for reviewing the administration of this policy. The Director–HR Compliance will periodically monitor compliance to this policy.

E. Noncompliance with the Policy
Noncompliance with the policy is handled in accordance with *Personnel Policies for Staff Members 61, 62, 63, 64, 65, and 67*, pertaining to disciplinary and separation matters.

V. PROCEDURES

A. Lactation Facilities

The University will provide a locked, private space that is sanitary--including appropriate temperature and ventilation--and equipped with a table, comfortable chair, and electrical outlet. If possible, the lactation space either will be located near a source of running water or will have a sink with running water in it.

The space will be in close proximity to the nursing mother's work area, generally not more than a 5-7 minute walk.

Appropriate lactation facilities include, but are not limited to, the employee's private office, another private office not in use, a conference room that can be secured, a multi-purpose room, or any available space with a locking door that is shielded from view and free from intrusion from co-workers, students, and the public.

Restrooms, spaces lacking privacy, or spaces lacking a locking door are not considered appropriate spaces for lactation purposes. However, an anteroom or lounge area connected to a restroom may be sufficient if the space is private, free from intrusion, and can be locked and shielded from view.

B. Accommodation Requests

A nursing mother is encouraged to discuss her needs, in terms of accommodations as well as the frequency and timing of breaks, with her supervisor. These shared discussions will help nursing mothers and supervisors arrange for mutually agreeable break times, typically 2-3 times a day.

A supervisor who receives a lactation accommodation request will work, as needed, with a Human Resources representative or the location's breastfeeding support program representative to identify available appropriate space and determine a break schedule. Break schedules should be based on the needs of a nursing mother and the operational considerations of the University.

C. Recourse

An employee who has comments, concerns, or questions regarding the University's Policy On Accommodations for Nursing Mothers should contact the local Human Resources Office or the location's breastfeeding support program.

A nursing mother who believes she has been denied appropriate accommodation should contact her local Human Resources Office.

VI. RELATED INFORMATION

- _Personnel Policies for Staff Members 31 (Hours of Work)_ (referenced in Section III.B of this policy)
- _California Fair Employment and Housing Act, Government Code Section 12926_
- _California Family Rights Act, Government Code Section 12945_
- _California Labor Code Section 1030-1033_

- *Fair Labor Standards Act – 29 U.S.C 207.r.1*
- *Patient Protection and Affordable Care Act – Section 4207 (Reasonable Break Time for Nursing Mothers)*
- *U.S. Department of Health and Human Services Agency – The Business Case for Breastfeeding*
- *Personnel Policies for Staff Members 2 (Definition of Terms)*
- *Personnel Policies for Staff Members 2.210 (Absence from Work)*
- *Personnel Policies for Staff Members 81 (Reasonable Accommodation)*
- *Lawrence Berkeley National Laboratory – For Nursing Mothers*
- *UC Berkeley – Breastfeeding Support Program*
- *UC Davis – Breastfeeding Support Program*
- *UC Irvine – Lactation Accommodation Guidelines*
- *UC Los Angeles – Lactation Accommodation Procedures*
- *UC Merced – Lactation Accommodation*
- *UC Office of the President – Lactation Program for New Mothers*
- *UC Riverside – Lactation Accommodation Program*
- *UC San Diego – Lactation Accommodation Policy*
- *UC San Francisco – Breastfeeding Services*
- *UC Santa Barbara – Breastfeeding Support Program*
- UC Santa Cruz – Breastfeeding Guidelines [under development]

VII. FREQUENTLY ASKED QUESTIONS

1. What is considered a reasonable lactation break?
Generally, nursing mothers need 2-3 lactation breaks during an 8-hour work period. A reasonable amount of time for a lactation break generally will not exceed 30 minutes per break and includes the time associated with travel to and from the lactation space, expressing milk, clean up, and storage.

2. Will a refrigerator for storing milk be provided by the University?
When feasible, yes.

3. How will the University plan for new lactation facilities or for improving current ones? New building plans as well as plans for renovating existing University buildings should consider the need for inclusion of appropriate lactation facilities. UC can lead the way in taking lactation accommodation from simply accommodation to truly best practices.

VIII. REVISION HISTORY

This is a new policy and has no revision history.

Establishing a Mother's Room

An integral part of the Breastfeeding Support Program is finding physical space on Johns Hopkins campuses to support the needs of mothers who breastfeed. As a result, the Breastfeeding Support Program has established several Mother's Rooms and plans to partner with other managers to open more.

What is a Mother's Room and why is it necessary?

A Mother's Room can best be described as a physical space that provides a clean, private, and comfortable place for women to express breast milk.

Expressing milk is a biological function that is aided by women being relaxed and comfortable. Often a cluttered office with ringing phones and knocks on the door will not provide the ideal atmosphere for quickly and efficiently expressing milk.

At a minimum, the room should:

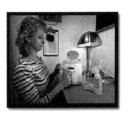

- assure privacy
- provide electricity for a breast pump
- have adequate lighting and ventilation
- be accessible to employees with disabilities
- include a table and comfortable chair
- provide appropriate hand washing and cleaning supplies

Ideally, a Mother's Room is centrally located and provides the following:

- a sink or close proximity to a sink
- a refrigerator
- separate temperature control
- a hospital-grade pump*
- a nursing stool
- attractive décor

* The Office of Work, Life and Engagement will provide a breast pump for fully-dedicated Mother's Rooms (See the Mother's Room Agreement, page 9, for more information.)

Mother's Rooms must be stocked with supplies at all times. At minimum, supplies include:

- hand sanitizer
- disposable towels
- latex gloves
- dishwashing detergent
- disinfecting wipes

Adapted from the Centers for Disease Control and Prevention Healthier Worksite Initiative (http://www.cdc.gov/nccdphp/dnpao/hwi/toolkits/lactation/planning.htm)

Johns Hopkins Office of Work, Life and Engagement | Breastfeeding Support Program | 09/15/2012

JH MOTHER'S ROOM AGREEMENT FORM

Supporting breastfeeding mothers is a shared responsibility. The Mother's Room Agreement details the responsibilities of the Office of Work, Life and Engagement, Mother's Room Owner, and Mother's Room User.

Office of Work, Life and Engagement/Benefits agrees to:

- Maintain a section of the Work, Life and Engagement website to provide employees with information about available breastfeeding support services and educational resources
- Maintain a list of Mother's Rooms on the Johns Hopkins campuses and their contact persons
- Provide hospital-grade breast pump(s) for Mother's Rooms that are:
  - in compliance with the law
  - secure
  - used primarily for expressing breast milk
- Give Mother's Room owners an orientation to hospital-grade breast pumps
- Provide materials for Mother's Room users about the proper use and cleaning of hospital-grade breast pumps
- Maintain an online registration process for Mother's Room users
- Provide blank sign-in sheets to Mother's Room Owners and track utilization of Mother's Rooms
- Provide promotional materials to Mother's Room Owners regarding work-life benefits

Mother's Room Owner agrees to:

- Arrange for Facilities department to secure the hospital-grade breast pump(s) to a stationery object
- Ensure that there is a functioning lock on the Mother's Room door
- Arrange for registered users to receive a key or key code for the door (if applicable)
- Give WorkLife staff access to the Mother's Room
- Provide furnishings (e.g. chair, table, and wall decorations)
- Ensure that the Mother's Room is cleaned regularly, including regular trash removal
- Purchase and stock supplies (disinfecting wipes, rubber gloves, hand soap, dishwashing soap, and paper towels)
- Display promotional materials provided by the Office of Work, Life and Engagement
- Provide completed sign-in sheet(s) to Office of Work, Life and Engagement monthly

Mother's Room User agrees to:

- Register with the Office of Work, Life and Engagement to use a Mother's Room
- Attend orientation (in person or online)
- Comply with registration and sign-in procedures
- Purchase an accessory kit for a hospital-grade pump or bring personal breast pump
- Clean hospital-grade breast pump before and after each use

The Room Owner agrees to immediately share any concerns with the Office of Work, Life and Engagement so that they can be resolved swiftly. The Office of Work, Life and Engagement reserves the right to remove a hospital-grade pump if these guidelines are not followed or if there are no mother's currently using the breast pump.

_____   _____   _____
Room Owner Name (Print)   Title   Room

_____   _____
Room Owner Signature   Date

Johns Hopkins Office of Work, Life and Engagement | Breastfeeding Support Program | 09/15/2012

169

Johns Hopkins Hospital Policy

The JHH policy regarding reasonable break time for mothers who breastfeed states:

> Supervisors should make every reasonable accommodation to support the needs of nursing mothers, including permitting them to visit the lactation room during normal break times or meal times. While a supervisor may require the lactation break time, if feasible, to run concurrently with break times already provided, supervisors should be as flexible as possible in allowing nursing mothers to select appropriate times to utilize the lactation room. Employees should work with their supervisors to effectively schedule this break time. If necessary, managers should also allow reasonable unpaid time to nursing mothers who require additional time outside of normal break or meal times.

This statement is located in the Johns Hopkins Health System Corporation and The Johns Hopkins Hospital Human Resource Policy and Procedure Manual. XV, 2.e, on page 12.

http://hopkinsworklife.org/docs/pdfs/HR300_comp-HPO_Update_6-1-2012.pdf

Note: Mother's Rooms are lactation rooms.

Johns Hopkins University Policy

In keeping with the Fair Labor Standards Act, all female faculty, staff and student-employees who breastfeed their children (collectively referred to herein as "nursing mothers") will be provided reasonable break times to express milk throughout the day, each time they need to express milk, for as long as the employee has a need to express milk. The University will also provide appropriate private areas, other than bathrooms, for this purpose. The area provided, if not dedicated to the nursing mother's use, will be made available when needed by the employee. The area provided will be shielded from view, and free from any intrusion from co-workers and the public.

Nursing mothers who need to express milk during the working day should contact their supervisor, department administrator and/or Human Resources. Working with the nursing mother, the supervisor or departmental administrator is required to provide reasonable break times and to identify an appropriate location. If possible, break times may be taken during regularly scheduled meal and rest breaks.

Nursing mothers must be paid for short breaks (20 minutes or less) otherwise given to employees. If the nursing mother is a non-exempt (hourly) employee and her breaks exceeds 20 minutes, her supervisor should make a good faith effort to permit the nursing mother to make up time. If no reasonable opportunity exists for a non-exempt nursing mother to make up time, a break time in excess of 20 minutes will not be paid. Nursing mothers who are exempt under the FLSA will not have pay docked for taking a break to express milk.

Questions regarding this policy may be addressed to the appropriate divisional Human Resources office.

Effective: December 29, 2011

http://web.jhu.edu/administration/jhuoie/docs/Resources-Policies/JHU%20Policy%20Regarding%20Reasonable%20Break%20Time%20for%20Nursing%20Mothers.pdf

JH BREASTFEEDING SUPPORT PROGRAM
REGISTRATION FORM

Name

JHED ID

Email

Daytime Phone

JH Affiliation   ☐ JHH/ JHHSC   ☐ JHU

DOB of Baby or Baby's Due Date (mm/dd/yyyy)

Anticipated Date of Return to Work (mm/dd/yyyy)

Indicate the Mother's Room(s) that you plan to use:

☐ Nelson Building, Room 134   ☐ OHS in Wyman Park Building

☐ Harriet Lane/Rubenstein Building   ☐ Keswick

☐ CRB II   ☐ Other

Is this your first experience with breastfeeding?

☐ Yes   ☐ No

Is this your first experience with pumping?

☐ Yes   ☐ No

Do you own a personal breast pump?

☐ Yes   ☐ No

You may be eligible for a free accessory kit for a hospital-grade pump supplied by the Office of Work, Life and Engagement if you earn less than $40,000 a year.

☐ Please check this box if you are interested in receiving an accessory pump kit.

Would you like to attend a Back to Work Breastfeeding Class?

☐ Yes   ☐ No

How did you learn about the Breastfeeding Support Program?

[Submit by Email]

JOHNS HOPKINS

WORK, *Life*
and Engagement

Mother's
Room

Open to Johns Hopkins faculty, staff and employees

Breastfeeding Support Program
443-997-7000
www.hopkinsworklife.org/breastfeeding

JOHNS HOPKINS

WORK, *Life*
and Engagement

Welcome!

Johns Hopkins recognizes the positive benefits of breastfeeding for both you and your child. The Breastfeeding Support Program is here to help so that you can breastfeed for as long as it is the best choice for you and your baby.

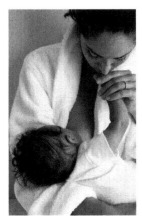

Questions, comments or suggestions?
Contact Meg Stoltzfus at worklife@jhu.edu or
443-997-7000.

Breastfeeding Support Program

www.hopkinsworklife.org/breastfeeding

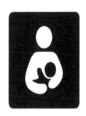

Brought to you at no cost as part of your HR benefits package

WORK, *Life* and Engagement

JOHNS HOPKINS

Breastfeeding Support Program

www.hopkinsworklife.org/breastfeeding

443-997-7000

Johns Hopkins Supports Mothers who Breastfeed

- Mother's Rooms on multiple campuses

- Breastfeeding classes

- Community and online breastfeeding resources

- Baby Shower to prepare expecting parents

- Child care referrals and backup care information

- Resources for managers

Contact worklife@jhu.edu or 443-997-7000 for more information.

It's the Law

State Law

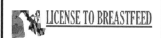

LICENSE TO BREASTFEED

Maryland Law: Health - General, § 20-801

A mother may breastfeed her child in any public or private location in which the mother and child are authorized to be. A person may not restrict or limit the right of a mother to breastfeed her child.

www.marylandbreastfeedingcoalition.org

Federal Law

LICENSE TO BREASTPUMP

Federal Law: Health Care Reform §4207

An employer shall provide a reasonable **break time** for an employee to express breast milk for her nursing child for 1 year after the child's birth, and a **place, other than a bathroom,** which may be used by an employee to express breast milk.

www.marylandbreastfeedingcoalition.org

JH TRACKING SPREADSHEET

Johns Hopkins Breastfeeding Support Program: Total Usage for First Half of FY13

Division	July		August		September		October		November		December	
JHU	Users	Visits	Users	Visits	Users	Visits	Users	Visits	Users	Visits	Users	Visits
Faculty	14	115	13	118	12	104	8	100	11	56	5	31
Staff	14	243	18	378	16	318	23	346	22	401	23	340
Total	28	358	31	496	28	422	31	446	33	457	28	371
JHU (in training)	Users	Visits	Users	Visits	Users	Visits	Users	Visits	Users	Visits	Users	Visits
Post Docs	13	213	13	266	20	376	23	390	22	349	25	298
Residents	5	32	4	19	5	20	3	87	4	87	6	79
Grad Students	15	272	14	251	10	170	12	125	7	83	5	51
Total	33	517	31	536	35	566	38	602	33	519	36	428
JHH/S	Users	Visits	Users	Visits	Users	Visits	Users	Visits	Users	Visits	Users	Visits
Employees	35	456	37	487	34	427	46	589	38	488	31	477
Total	35	456	38	489	34	427	46	589	38	488	31	477
Overall Total	*96*	*1331*	*100*	*1521*	*97*	*1415*	*115*	*1637*	*104*	*1464*	*95*	*1276*

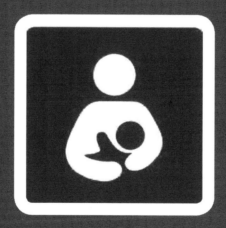

PRIVACY PLEASE
MOTHER AT WORK

Johns Hopkins Office of Work, Life and Engagement
www.hopkinsworklife.org/breastfeeding

JOHNS HOPKINS SUPPORTS BREASTFEEDING

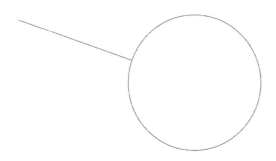

Johns Hopkins is committed to providing mothers with information and support if they choose to breastfeed after returning to work.

Experts agree that breastfeeding **improves** the health of mothers and babies.

The U.S. Surgeon General **encourages** active involvement and support from family members, friends, communities, clinicians, health care systems, and employers to make breastfeeding easier.

Federal law **requires** employers to provide break time and a clean, private place to express breast milk.

Johns Hopkins Breastfeeding Support Program components:

- Mother's Rooms with hospital-grade breast pumps
- Online resources for employees and managers
- Discounted breast pumps for purchase
- Baby Shower and other WorkLife services to assist new parents

Johns Hopkins Breastfeeding Support Program
For more information, visit
www.hopkinsworklife.org/breastfeeding,
call 443-997-7000, or email worklife@jhu.edu.

JOHNS HOPKINS SUPPORTS BREASTFEEDING

Resources

Academy of Breastfeeding Medicine: www.bfmed.org

Affordable Care Act: www.healthcare.gov/

American Academy of Pediatrics: www.aap.org

American Public Health Association Maternal Child Health Section: www.apha.org

Break Time for Nursing Mothers: www.dol.org

Business Case for Breastfeeding: www.everymother.org/workplace/view/index.php

Breastfeeding USA: breastfeedingusa.org

College and University Work-Life-Family Association: www.cuwfa.org

Connecticut Breastfeeding Coalition: www.breastfeedingCT.org

CDC: www.cdc.gov [state report cards at www.cdc.gov/breastfeeding/data/reportcard.htm]

Family and Medical Leave Act: www.dol.org

George Washington University: parentinginitiative.gwu.edu/

Healthy People 2020 Topics and Objectives, Maternal and Infant Health: www.healthypeople.gov

International Board of Lactation Consultant Examiners: www.iblce.org

International Lactation Consultants Association: www.ilca.org

It's Only Natural Campaign: www.womenshealth.gov/itsonlynatural/

Johns Hopkins University: www.hopkinsworklife.org/services/breastfeeding/index.html

La Leche League International: www.llli.org

Let's Move Campaign: www.letsmove.gov

Michigan State University: www.frc.msu.edu/Parents/Breastfeeding.htm

University of Arizona: lifework.arizona.edu/cc/lactation_information

University of California Davis: worklife-wellness.ucdavis.edu/

University of Rhode Island: www.uri.edu/advance/work_life_support/lactation_facilities.html

U.S. Breastfeeding Committee: www.usbreastfeeding.org/

U.S Office of Minority Health: minorityhealth.hhs.gov

U.S. Office on Women's Health Breastfeeding: www.womenshealth.gov

U.S. Surgeon General's Call to Support Breastfeeding: www.surgeongeneral.gov/library/calls/breastfeeding/

WIC: www.fns.usda.gov/wic/Breastfeeding/breastfeeding

Index

T

Technology 147
Telecommuting 37, 48, 51, 120
Tracking Usage 130

U

University of Arizona 25, 93, 99,
        100, 103, 104, 191, 194
University of California Davis 24,
        77, 144, 146, 189
University of Michigan 143, 146
University of Rhode Island 24, 59,
        67, 145, 147, 148

V

Vending Machine 26, 138, 142,
        147
Vision of Excellence 24, 78, 79,
        82

W

World Health Organization 50, 57

Contributing Authors

Barbara A. Ashby, MS, WLCP

As Manager of WorkLife and Wellness at the University of California Davis, Barbara Ashby has devoted her career and community service to program and policy development supporting children and families. A Work-Life Certified Professional, Ms. Ashby has nearly 30 years of experience in research, teaching, and human services. Her work has earned the Innovative Excellence Award from the Alliance of Work/Life Professionals, the Family Services Award from the Orfalea Family Foundation, Mother-Baby Friendly Workplace awards from the Breastfeeding Coalition of Yolo County and The California Task Force on Youth and Workplace Wellness, and the AWLP Work-Life Seal of Distinction. Most recently, the UC Davis Breastfeeding Support Program, which she founded, was selected by the U.S. Department of Health and Human Services Office on Women's Health as a model for lactation accommodation in higher education.

Ms. Ashby holds a Bachelor's degree in Psycholinguistics from Brown University, Master's in Child Development from UC Davis, and a California Community College Teaching Credential. She is a member of the College and University Work Family Association, National Coalition for Campus Children's Centers, and AWLP/WorldatWork. She was selected as a WorkLife Rising Star during the inaugural year of the award, subsequently served on the AWLP/WorldatWork Strategy Board, and advocates locally and nationally for work-life effectiveness.

On the home front, Barbara's approach to wellness centers on yoga, walking, gardening, and a bevy of pets. She is the mother of two breastfed daughters and grandmother of two breastfed grandchildren.

Michelle Carlstrom

Michelle Carlstrom is the Senior Director of the Office of Work, Life and Engagement, serving both Johns Hopkins University and the Johns Hopkins Health System and Hospital. Michelle holds a Master's Degree in Social Work, with a specialization in Employee Assistance. She has worked as both a counselor and administrator in the E.A.P. and WorkLife fields for nearly twenty years. She has extensive training experience in workplace behavioral health and wellness programs, delivering tailored services to groups of employees. Michelle is a regular consultant to human resource professionals and other management executives on areas of stress management, work-life balance, and managing at-risk employees. She has worked with and provided training to a variety of companies, including government agencies, non-profit organizations, and Fortune 500 companies. In her current role at Johns Hopkins, she leads an office that delivers services and programs to assist nearly 45,000 employees through the challenging intersections of work and life, with a focus on keeping people engaged in the workplace and the surrounding community. Included in these services is the Johns Hopkins Breastfeeding Support Program.

Cathy Carothers, BLA, IBCLC, FILCA

Cathy Carothers is co-director of EVERY MOTHER, INC., a non-profit organization providing counseling and lactation training for health professionals across the United States. She is immediate past Chair of the United States Breastfeeding Committee, and past president of the International Lactation Consultant Association. She is a Fellow of ILCA, and has been an International Board Certified Lactation Consultant since 1996.

Cathy is the author of the national HHS Maternal and Child Health Bureau project, *The Business Case for Breastfeeding,* and served as lead trainer and technical assistance consultant for the national training initiative in 36 U.S. states. She currently serves as project director for the national HHS Office on Women's Health initiative, "Supporting Nursing Moms at Work: Employer Solutions," to assist employers of hourly workers with worksite lactation accommodations as part of the Affordable Care Act. She also worked with New York State Department of Health to develop a statewide worksite initiative, including the toolkit, "Making it Work." Cathy works extensively with business organizations and labor unions to provide education and support for accommodating breastfeeding women at work.

An experienced trainer and speaker, Cathy has provided more than 400 training events in every U.S. state and territory, and several countries. She is the project director for other national breastfeeding programs for the Federal government, including the breastfeeding peer counseling program for the USDA WIC Program, *Loving Support Through Peer Counseling: A Journey Together,* and the national WIC staff curriculum in breastfeeding, *Using Loving Support to Grow and Glow in WIC.* A former University public relations director, she served as the State Breastfeeding Coordinator for the Mississippi WIC Program, coordinating the state's comprehensive peer counseling program and breastfeeding promotion campaign that earned them the "National WIC Award."

Cathy is married to a United Methodist minister, and is the mother of five healthy breastfed children, now ages 22 to 33. She is also the proud grandmother to two beautiful breastfed grandsons, ages four and two.

Erica Hayton, MPH

Erica Hayton, Director of Benefits & Wellness at the George Washington University (GW), has led GW's work-life and wellness program since 2007. During this time Erica has grown the program from a small, part-time initiative to a key component of GW's overall HR strategy, with a dedicated team of work-life professionals. Erica also serves on the Board of Directors for the College and University Work-Life-Family Association, on the steering committee for her local World at Work Work-Life Network, and is an adjunct faculty member in GW's School of Public Health and Health Services, teaching "Workplace Health Promotion."

Caryn Jung, MS

Caryn Jung coordinates the University of Arizona's (UA) nationally recognized childcare (including lactation resources), eldercare, and work-life programs at Life & Work Connections (LWC). These LWC programs serve faculty, staff, and students at the state's only land-grant university.

Caryn's contributions involve the expansion of UA's Lactation Resources and Sick Child and Emergency/Back-Up Care Program, and the development of the "Flexible Work Arrangements Guide." The UA's first eldercare specialist, her career reflects a life cycle philosophy that encourages personal and organizational resiliency. She holds a Master of Science degree in gerontology and a Bachelor's degree in child development.

A work-life educator and practitioner in higher education, healthcare, and non-profit fields, Caryn directs diverse knowledge and experience in early childhood care and education, gerontology, eldercare and caregiving, and flexible work arrangements to develop initiatives that support individual and organizational recruitment and retention efforts for a multi-generational workforce and student body.

Caryn has been recognized for campus leadership and volunteer efforts, presents and writes on topics of work and life integration, and is a chapter co-author in "*Establishing The Family-Friendly Campus: Models for Effective Practice.*" Professional board and member experiences include the City of Los Angeles Mayor's Advisory Committee on Child Care and Vice President of the College and University Work-Life-Family Association (CUWFA).

Caryn modeled lactation best practice approaches with her own family. She continues to promote the maternal and child health benefits of lactation and facilitate the growth of lactation resources as an effective work-life strategy within her institution and the work-life field.

Ian Reynolds

Ian Reynolds is Director of WorkLife and Community Programs in the Office of Work, Life and Engagement at Johns Hopkins. In his position Ian oversees the delivery of a variety of programs designed to assist faculty and staff achieve healthy work-life effectiveness. These include the Breastfeeding Support Program; lifespan workshops; childcare, backup care, and eldercare services; flexible work arrangements; staff recognition; and housing and relocation support. Ian also directs a number of community outreach efforts, which include an annual United Way Campaign, Red Cross blood drives, professional clothing drives, holiday donation programs to benefit families and seniors in need, and the Johns Hopkins Takes Time for Schools volunteer program. Prior to assuming his current role in 2011, Ian worked for 11 years at the Johns Hopkins Center for Talented Youth where he most recently held the position of Director of Family Academic Programs. He received his M.A. in American Studies from the University of Wyoming. Ian lives in Columbia with his wife Stephanie and their three boys, all of whom were breastfed. A benefit to the health of all three children, breastfeeding was especially important for their youngest son who was born with Down syndrome and had additional health concerns.

Barb Silver

Barb Silver is a Research Professor in Psychology and the Research Coordinator at the Schmidt Labor Research Center (SLRC) at the University of Rhode Island. She has focused her research interests on gender, in particular women's career advancement. At URI from 2003-2009, she directed a $3.5 million National Science Foundation ADVANCE program to recruit, retain, and foster the careers of women faculty in science and engineering, including work-life policy and program development. In 2007, through an Elsevier Foundation grant, she created an award-winning model lactation program at the University for new mothers returning to work. Currently, as Research Coordinator at the SLRC, Silver is focusing her research and policy work on work-life balance and workplace flexibility. For the past ten years, she has co-chaired the URI Work-Life Committee, which has been active in promoting policy development, workshops, and education around the issues of work-life balance and workplace flexibility at URI. She has taught courses in Psychology and Women's Studies, has served as an outside consultant and workshop facilitator on regional campuses, and has presented at many conferences on issues of work-life, gender equity, diversity, mentoring, and workplace flexibility. She is the proud mother of two breastfed daughters.

Meg Stoltzfus, M.S.

Meg Stoltzfus is the Lifespan Services Manager in the Office of Work, Life and Engagement at Johns Hopkins. In this role Meg helps employees plan for family transitions and investigate care-giving resources across the lifespan. She develops programs and facilitates workshops for employees, such as breastfeeding support, parenting strategies, services for aging adults, and coping with stress in order to help Johns Hopkins employees engage more fully in both work and life. Meg has developed a program to assist pre-retirees in preparing for the transition to retirement and coordinates programs and services for JHU retirees. She received her M.S. in counseling in 1999 from the University of North Carolina at Greensboro and is a Licensed Clinical Professional Counselor in Maryland. Meg earned a certificate in Geriatric Care Management in 2011. She lives in Baltimore with her husband and her two breastfed children.

Lori Strom

Lori Strom graduated from the University of Oregon with a Bachelor's Degree in Community Services and Public Affairs with a focus on Gerontology in 1978. In 1990 she received a Master's Degree in Public Administration with a focus on Healthcare from Western Michigan University.

Lori has been the Coordinator of the Michigan State University Family Resource Center since 1997. The Family Resource Center provides services and resources to assist MSU faculty, staff, and students in their balance of work, educational, and family responsibilities. Services include free Emergency Backup Childcare, subsidized Sick Childcare, free access to web-based caregivers and more. Lori has acquired millions of dollars in childcare grants to subsidize the cost of childcare for low-income students, in addition to other student-parent support services to enable them to persist and graduate.

Since Lori has been a breastfeeding mother of two sons, she understands the importance of breastfeeding support in the workplace. She established the MSU Breastfeeding Support Service in the Family Resource Center in 2000. The FRC office consults with moms, produces the brochure, maintains the breastfeeding website, and updates the rooms on the Google Map on behalf of nursing mothers. The FRC sponsors the breastfeeding class series and hosts the breastfeeding email listserv. Lori teaches seminars on flexibility, convened the Flex for U committee that encouraged the importance of flexible work arrangements across campus, and consults with employees and supervisors on how to implement flexible schedules.

Jan Sturges, M.Ed., LPC

Jan Sturges has an extensive career in not-for-profit organizational management, with an emphasis in healthcare administration and gerontology. Jan is also an educator, eldercare consultant, and public speaker on topics related to aging, healthcare, and life cycle issues. She received her Master's of Education Degree in Counseling and Guidance from the University of Arizona in 1986, and is licensed as a professional counselor by the Arizona Board of Behavioral Health Examiners.

Currently, Jan is the Caregiving Coordinator for the University of Arizona, Life & Work Connections, Eldercare and Life Cycle Resources. In this role she provides resource information and consultation support to faculty, staff, and students who are caregivers for dependent individuals and older adults. She also conducts workshops on caregiving, dependent care strategies, and life transitions throughout the life cycle.

Earlier in Jan's 27-year career, she developed, implemented, and managed a multi-faceted senior wellness program at Tucson Medical Center that served more than 22,000 older adults throughout Southern Arizona. As a specialist in the field of aging, health, and dependent-care issues, Jan was a co-host of *People Plus*, a local television program devoted to healthcare and aging topics. As founder and President of the Caregiver Consortium, a non-profit organization that provides educational programs for family caregivers, Jan produced a resource guide, *How to Be a Resilient Caregiver*, which was funded by United Way of Tucson and Southern Arizona in collaboration with the Caregiver Consortium. The guide has been widely distributed to more than 20,000 caregivers in Southern Arizona and is available online through several healthcare-related websites, including UA Life & Work Connections.

Darci Thompson, MSW, LCSW, SPHR

Darci Thompson is the Director of UA Life & Work Connections (LWC) at the University of Arizona (UA). Unique features of this program address "whole person wellness" through the integration of employee assistance, worksite wellness, child and eldercare services, and work-life support to more than 14,000 faculty and staff. Select dependent care services are also provided to students. These combined efforts provide a unique life cycle response that enhances employee/student wellbeing and retention.

As a licensed clinical social worker, Darci has more than 20 years of clinical, managerial, and work-life experience. She applies a work-life perspective when educating supervisors and employees on achieving resilience, promoting wellness, and mitigating risk in the academic/work environment. She presents to national, state, and local forums, serves as an external consultant/educator, research associate, and a faculty associate of the Arizona State University School of Social Work, and is certified as a Senior Professional in Human Resources by the Society for Human Resources Management. Darci holds a Master of Social Work degree and is a chapter co-author in "*Journal of Workplace Behavioral Health,*" "*The Integration of Employee Assistance, Work/Life, and Wellness Services,*" and "*Establishing The Family-Friendly Campus: Models for Effective Practice.*"

About the Editors

Michele K. Griswold, MPH, RN, IBCLC

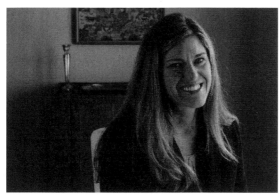

Michele K. Griswold has almost 20 years experience working with mothers and children, both clinically and in public health. She was a founding member of the Connecticut Breastfeeding Coalition (CBC) and is the current Chairperson. Her work with the coalition includes experience in planning and implementing breastfeeding programs in the hospital setting and in the workplace setting. Specifically, she has experience presenting and implementing *The Business Case for Breastfeeding* to employers on a statewide level. Under her leadership, she oversaw the disbursement of federal funding to 11 Connecticut employers to implement "The Business Case." Eight of those employers were public schools and one was a university. As the Chair of the CBC, she often lectures to students, community activists, and other stakeholders. She has represented Connecticut to the U.S. Breastfeeding Committee's National Meeting of State and Tribal Coalitions three times. Her advocacy experience is diverse and includes collaborative work with governmental agencies and legislators.

Michele has been a registered nurse for 25 years and an International Board Certified Lactation Consultant since 2001. She has been actively involved in the International Lactation Consultant Association (ILCA) through work with the Accreditation Task Force that led to the establishment of LAARC, the body that provides oversight of education for the profession. She is currently Chair of the Global Outreach Committee for ILCA, and one of ILCA's liaisons to the United Nations. She is also a doctoral student at the University of Massachusetts, Graduate School of Nursing, Worcester. As a working and former nursing mother, she is passionate about innovative ways to overcome barriers for breastfeeding families.

Michele L. Vancour, Ph.D., MPH

Michele L. Vancour is a past president of the College and University Work-Life-Family Association (CUWFA). In this capacity she oversaw several works that present best practices in the work-life field focusing on higher education, and can attest that one of the most commonly sought topics for information is lactation on campus. She is a member of the Connecticut Breastfeeding Coalition's (CBC) Board of Directors, responsible for overseeing breastfeeding research, and has helped the CBC identify best practices in lactation support in various work settings across Connecticut. Michele is committed to building the future capacity of breastfeeding public health 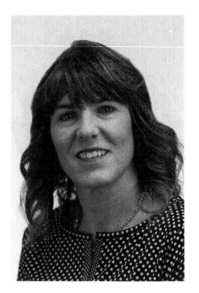 experts through her mentorship of public health interns working with the CBC, as well as encouraging students to focus their research on breastfeeding-related issues.

Michele is a professor of public health at Southern Connecticut State University (SCSU). She teaches maternal and child health and health promotion courses. In 2001, she began conducting research highlighting academic women's struggles with breastfeeding once they returned to their campus positions after the birth of their children. Her research findings resulted in the establishment of SCSU's lactation room and support program. Further, she has published and presented on the topic of breastfeeding in higher education. She is proud to have successfully balanced her academic career while raising two breastfed boys.

Dear Reader,

Thank you for purchasing and reading this book. You can find more information about the book on our website: www.academicbreastfeeding.com.

If you found our book helpful, please consider writing a review of the book on our website, Amazon.com, HalePublishing.com, and/or on any other appropriate websites.

Sincerely,

Editors, *Breastfeeding Best Practices in Higher Education*

Ordering Information

Hale Publishing, L.P.
1825 E Plano Parkway, Suite 280
Plano, Texas, USA 75074

8:00 am to 5:00 pm CST

Call » 972-578-0400
Toll free » 800.378.1317
Fax » 972-578-0413

Online
www.HalePublishing.com